Devices for Mobility and Manipulation for People with Reduced Abilities

REHABILITATION SCIENCE IN PRACTICE SERIES

Series Editors

Marcia J. Scherer, Ph.D.

President
Institute for Matching Person and Technology

Professor
Orthopaedics and Rehabilitation
University of Rochester Medical Center

Dave Muller, Ph.D.

Executive
Suffolk New College

Editor-in-Chief
Disability and Rehabilitation

Founding Editor
Aphasiology

Devices for Mobility and Manipulation for People with Reduced Abilities

Teodiano Freire Bastos-Filho
Federal University of Espirito Santo, Vitoria, Brazil

Dinesh Kumar
RMIT University, Melbourne, Australia

Sridhar Poosapadi Arjunan
RMIT University, Melbourne, Australia

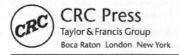

CRC Press
Taylor & Francis Group
Boca Raton London New York

CRC Press is an imprint of the
Taylor & Francis Group, an **informa** business

CRC Press
Taylor & Francis Group
6000 Broken Sound Parkway NW, Suite 300
Boca Raton, FL 33487-2742

First issued in paperback 2017

Version Date: 20140320

ISBN 13: 978-1-4665-8645-1 (hbk)
ISBN 13: 978-1-138-07378-4 (pbk)

Visit the Taylor & Francis Web site at
http://www.taylorandfrancis.com

and the CRC Press Web site at
http://www.crcpress.com

Contents

List of Tables

List of Figures

Foreword

A few years ago, we started the Biosignals and Biorobotics Conference (IEEE BRC). The theme of the conference was affordable healthcare and assistive devices. One of our observations was that there was a significant difference between the technology and devices that were available in the laboratories and those available to the users. While this is common for all technologies, we observed that this difference was more in assistive technologies, perhaps because the users had become resigned to their reduced abilities. Thus, we realised the need for a book that would help bridge the gap and disseminate the research outcomes of the laboratories to non-technical people.

Sharing the research outcomes helps improve the visibility of the assistive technologies that are developed in laboratories. This is important for the users who gain access to a wider range of technologies and who get the benefit of new research and development. It will also help the scientists to showcase their research and be able to see the devices being used by the people who need them the most. It will help maximise the benefit of the research and innovation dollar that is generally spent by governments.

However, this ambition of authoring a book that discusses innovations in assistive technologies soon became more challenging than earlier anticipated. No two people are identical, and their needs are not the same. Thus, developing technology that will be useful for all people is always a challenge. However, when the target is those people who have lost the use of one or more of their limbs, this challenge is many times bigger. Not only are the levels of disability unique to the individual; their circumstances and aspirations are very different. Coupled with this is the significant difference in the social support that is available for the person. People in different societies receive different levels of support from their friends and family, and there is also a significant difference in the financial and medical support that is available to people who have reduced abilities of their limbs. Thus, with this background, we would like to introduce this book. We realise that it is impossible for any book on this topic to be complete and suitable for all people. However, we have used the philosophy 'Maximum benefit for maximum people.'

The target audience for this book is technical people who work with assistive technology, but also for the lay, non-technical people who may find technical jargon, equations and software details cumbersome and confusing. For their sake, we have attempted to keep some technical details away from part of the text, though we have provided a brief flavour when describing a specific example. We have provided the references for scientists, designers and others interested in the details so that they can easily access such details from the scientific papers. We are also aware that this field is rapidly evolving, and new devices and technologies are continually emerging.

One challenge when working with or developing assistive technology is the necessity for the team to be multidisciplinary. Over the years, we have observed that people from different disciplines communicate very differently. They use a different vocabulary with unique jargon, and express themselves differently. We have attempted to use plain language to make this book accessible to a wide range of professionals and lay people.

We would like to thank CNPq and CAPES (Brazil) for financial support, and RMIT University (Australia) and UFES (Brazil) for allowing us to work on this book. We would also like to thank all the collaborators of the book (students and colleagues) and the co-chairs of IEEE BRC who helped develop the ideas for this book. Without these supports, the book would not have been possible.

1

Introduction

Teodiano Freire Bastos-Filho
Universidade Federal do Espírito Santo, Brazil

Dinesh Kant Kumar
RMIT University, Australia

CONTENTS

1.1 Introduction

The global estimate of people who suffer and survive spinal cord injury (SCI) every year is 22 people/million inhabitants, or over 130,000 people each year worldwide [1]. In Australia, there are an estimated 241 SCI injuries/annum or the ratio of 13.2 people/million inhabitants; and in Brazil, according to [2], in 2010 there were 740,456 people in that condition. A majority of SCI patients become lifelong dependent on a wheelchair. The number of users of wheelchairs is significantly higher than people who have suffered SCI. Some of the causes for people to be unable to walk and require wheelchairs include amyotrophic lateral sclerosis (ALS) with 2 people per 100,000 per year, spinal cord tumor, cerebral palsy, multiple sclerosis, muscular distrophy (Duchenne and Becker), myasthenia gravis, and other diseases that affect the neuromuscular system. There are also those people who have lost their lower limbs due to disease, such as diabetes, or accidents, such as road trauma, or due to war and conflicts. And added to this list of people is the growing aging population who, due to age-associated weakness and loss of control, are unable to walk and commute unaided.

Medical advances have improved longevity for all humans, and reduced mortality due to trauma and disease, including people who have suffered neuromuscular or skeletal injuries. However, a number of these people who are alive due to advancement in medicine require the use of mobility devices, and thus, improved medical technologies have resulted in an increase in the number of people requiring assistance in their daily lives. With increased urbanization, nuclear families, and the fast pace of our lives, there is reduced support from family and friends, and people in many parts of the world require assistive technologies such as powered wheelchairs that can be used independently. Increased awareness due to the internet has also resulted in the changes of the aspirations and requirements of advanced features by patients and society in general. This has resulted in the need for greater advancements in technologies for assistive living.

1.2 Assistive Technology

Assistive technology devices (ATD) are any products, services, or devices that help people with reduced abilities to live their lives. The objective of ATDs is to improve the quality of life of individuals with disabilities (physical, sensing, or psychological) and help them to reduce their dependence on other people such as their caregivers, family, or friends, resulting in improved social inclusion and general well-being. One of the most important goals of the development and application of assistive technology is to minimize the social dependence of people with disabilities. Until quite recently, people from richer societies had the advantage of government services and support mechanisms for people with disabilities and were also the fortunate ones to obtain the assistive technologies. However, recent global financial and social changes have resulted in a much wider market for these devices.

There is a wide range of assistive technologies, from mobility devices such as wheelchairs and smart walkers to artificial hands, communication devices, and control interfaces to manage the surroundings. These devices range in complexity based on the level of support required by the patients. Different specialities contribute to the development of the assistive technology, such as engineering, architecture, design, education, psychology, occupational therapy, speech therapy, physiotherapy, medicine, and nursing. Specialists in these fields have further responsibilities in relation to their patients because their jobs are focused to make possible or improve a service to people with disabilities.

Significant improvements in fields such as materials, electronics, sensors, wireless communication, and computers have resulted in a new generation of robots, and this has resulted in the development of robotics for assistive purposes. These devices are smaller, lighter, stronger, and smarter than ever before. Low power consumption, wireless technologies, and smarter and faster processors have made these reliable and robust. These robotic devices have resulted in significant improvement in the quality of life of people with disabilities.

The main feature of assistive technologies is the user interface that ensures the convenience and reliability of the device, which is essential for safety, comfort, and functionality for the user. One common requirement for all advanced assistive devices is that these are computerized and require an effective and reliable way for the patient to interface with the device for giving the commands. Thus, an important aspect of such devices is the human–computer interface (HCI). The HCI for patients requiring assistive technologies has a wide range of complexities.

Some people who suffer from muscle weakness due to disease or old age may require the HCI to recognize their commands based on their low level of action or muscle contraction, which by itself may not be functionally effective. Individuals with motor impairments have difficulty executing movements or communicating with other people because the motor neurons that influence voluntary muscles are affected [5] [6]. On the other hand, some motor neuropathies, especially ALS, produce deformation and degeneration of muscular cells without affecting cognitive aspects [3] [5] [6] [8]. Thus, assistive technology can provide devices commanded by biomedical signals to help the mobility and maximize the ability to communicate for these people.

For some people, such as those in the early stages of a neuropathy such as ALS, the individuals have good finger touch control [6], making it possible to use touch screens to select commands, or a head pointer fixed on the user's head, as shown in Figure 1.1, or even a computer keyboard. However, due to the progression of the disease, or in patients with SCI, it is not always possible to use such interfaces. Thus, electrical

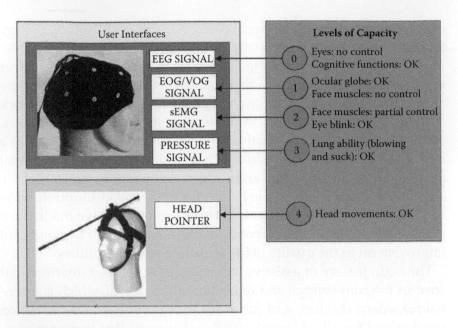

FIGURE 1.1
Signals adopted in different human–machine interfaces and the corresponding levels of capacity.
Adapted from [4].

signals from different parts of the human body have to be used as
command signals for controlling mechanical systems. However, it is
necessary that the individual in charge of controlling such devices be
able to intentionally generate such signals. It is also necessary that the
HCI adopted for this purpose can "understand" and process such signals reliably and in real time, setting the command that best fits the
wish of the individual. Figure 1.1 shows different kinds of signals according to the corresponding capacity levels of the user. The control
signal can be generated by eye blinks (myoelectric signal—sEMG),
eye movements (captured by facial electrodes—electrooculographic
signal, EOG—or through a video camera—videooculographic signal,
VOG), head or face movements (captured by an IMU—inertial measurement unit), blowing and sucking (sip and puff switch), and by
brain waves (electroencephalographic signals—EEG). This latter kind
of signal can be used for advanced stages of neuropathy because such
individuals may not have steady control of eye movements. In this situation, brain waves are the only possible source of biomedical signals.
Assistive devices can be broadly classified into three types: (i)
mobility devices such as wheelchairs and walkers, (ii) devices for

assistive learning, and (iii) manipulative devices such as prosthetic devices.

1.2.1 Mobility Devices: Wheelchairs and Walkers

Numerous people are unable to walk without assistance due to a range of ailments such as muscle weakness, lower-limb amputation, and inability to control their muscles. Although in the basic form, wheelchairs and walkers have been used for over 1,000 years, these have evolved over the past 30 years, and currently are able to provide self-determined and safe mobility for people who may not have control of any of their muscles. These are described in detail in Chapters 2, 3, 4, 5, and 6.

1.2.2 Devices for Assistive Learning

Children need to interact with their environment to develop their learning and cognition skills and for learning to interact with other children. However, physiological or psychological disorders may impair their learning abilities and this can result in lifelong difficulties. Devices have been developed that can assist children with overcoming some of these weakness. These devices assist children with special needs to interact with their environment through manipulation, leading to developing their learning and interaction skills. Often, functional assistance may also be incorporated in the same device. These devices are described in Chapter 7.

1.2.3 Prosthetic Devices

Prosthetic devices are essentially required by people who have suffered amputation of their limbs. While there may be multiple reasons for amputation of the limb of a person, the most common are (i) trauma and (ii) diabetes. Prosthetic devices range from user-powered mechanical devices to battery-powered and, more recently, robotic devices. The range of complexity and functionality varies significantly, from two-finger devices controlled by a switch, to the hand with four fingers and thumb that can be controlled by brain waves. Chapter 8 provides the details of the prosthetic hand.

References

[1] ICCP, *International campaign for cures of spinal cord injury paralysis.* http://www.campaignforcure.org, accessed May, 2012.

[2] *Brazilian 2010 Census 2010.* http://www.portaldeacessibilidade.rs. gov. br, accessed June 23, 2013.

[3] A S Brandao, D C Cavalieri, A Sa, T F Bastos-Filho, M Sarcinelli-Filho, *Controlling devices using biological signals.* Int J Adv Robot Syst, vol. 8, pp. 22–33, 2009.

[4] A Kubler, B Kotchoubey, J Kaiser, J R Wolpaw, N Birbaumer, *Brain computer communication: Unlocking the locked.* Psychol Bull, vol. 127 (3), pp. 358–375, 2001.

[5] J Hori, K Sakano, Y Saitoh, *Development of communication supporting device controlled by eye movements and voluntary eye blink.* Proceedings of Engineering in Medicine and Biology Society, IEMBS/IEEE, vol. 6, pp. 4302–4305, 2004.

[6] J B Polikoff, H T Bunnell, *Toward a P300-based computer interface.* RESNA '95 Annual Conference, vol. 1, pp. 178–180, 1995.

[7] R Barea, L Boquete, E López, M Mazo, *Guidance of a wheelchair using electrooculography.* CSCC/IEEE International Multiconference on Circuits, Systems, Communications and Computers, vol. 1, 1999.

[8] A Frizera-Neto, W C Celeste, V R Martins, T F Bastos-Filho, M Sarcinell-Filho, *Human-machine interface based on electro-biological signals for mobile vehicles.* Proceedings of International Symposium on Industrial Electronics, ISIE/IEEE, vol. 1, pp. 2954–2959, 2006.

2

Wheelchairs

Teodiano Freire Bastos-Filho
Universidade Federal do Espírito Santo, Brazil

Dinesh Kant Kumar
RMIT University, Australia

CONTENTS

2.1 History

A wheelchair is nothing but a chair with wheels and is designed to be a replacement for walking for people who are unable to walk. Images of wheeled chairs made specifically to carry people began to appear in Chinese art as early as 525 CE. While the use of wheelchairs grew during the Middle Ages, significant progress has taken place over the past five decades, and wheelchairs have since then evolved significantly.

2.2 Current Technologies

A typical wheelchair has four wheels, a seat, and handlebars located behind the seat that can be used for someone to push and maneuver the chair [1]. While in past years these wheelchairs were powered by the caregiver of the patient and were very useful for the patient, it confined the use to the few who could afford the luxury of employing a nurse or assistant. Subsequent advancements resulted in wheelchairs that were designed to allow the seated occupant to turn the rear wheels by hand and thus move and control the wheelchair independently. More recent developments have resulted in these wheelchairs being battery powered and propelled by motors with the help of an array of batteries that are typically located under the seat. Some of the very recent advancements have resulted in wheelchairs that are suitable for climbing stairs, such as the "TopChair" [2]. Improved materials have also resulted in the development of wheelchairs that are suitable for being used for sports and recreations, such as the chairs used during the Paralympic Games [3].

Wheelchairs are continuously evolving and now are not only catering to people who could not walk yet had strength and control of their upper limbs, but also to a range of people with different abilities and requirements. While one type of wheelchair users are people who do not have any strength and control in their lower or upper limbs, such as quadriplegics, and require significant assistance to control the wheelchair, the other end of the spectrum of users are those people who use the wheelchairs to play sports, go for hikes, and lead very normal lives and more. There are also those people such as the elderly, who require mobility devices due to weakness and fatigue. Thus, future wheelchairs need to be smart and often provide robotic capacities, and be equipped with sensors, computers, human–machine interfaces, advanced control systems, and safety for the users as well as the people in close proximity.

2.3 Technical Description and Specifications

Currently, wheelchairs can be divided into four categories. The first is the most commonly used wheelchair that requires manual manipulation, and may be propelled by the user or may be assisted by a caregiver. The second is the wheelchair that is motorized using a set of batteries. There are also the mobility scooters that are used by reasonably able people. Then there is the version that is suitable for athletes. These are manually operated by the user and allow increased levels of maneuverability and speed to the user. Each of these is described below.

2.3.1 Manual Wheelchair

2.3.1.1 System Description

This wheelchair is composed of a metallic tubing body with a cushioned seat and four wheels. The rear wheels are large, with a diameter ranging from 600 to 660 mm, and the front wheels (casters) are of a diameter ranging from 76 to 203 mm. The typical weight of these chairs is between 13 and 20 kg, able to carry a user up to approximately 113 kg, but there also exist heavy ones to carry users weighing from 160 to 200 kg. The overall typical dimensions are 610 to 760 mm (wide) and 1100 to 1500 mm (long). These chairs are made by many manufacturers, ranging from cottage industries to large manufacturers, and are often a subsidiary of cycle manufacturers. While most of these do not come with any safety mechanisms, some of these are provided with seat belts, extra cushioning, and support for the legs of the patients.

2.3.1.2 User Requirements

Manual wheelchairs can only be used by people who have upper limb strength or who are able to get the help from a nurse or caregiver.

2.3.1.3 User Benefits

The biggest benefit of manual wheelchairs is the cost and easy availability. These chairs are available in remote parts of the world, and cost in the range of US$200 and US$1,000. Manual wheelchairs are essential for people who have lost the ability to use their lower limbs. People who have lost their lower limbs due to amputation and have good strength and control of their upper limbs are able to use these chairs very effectively. These chairs are also extensively used by people who require temporary help, such as people who have fractured their lower limbs and are unable to walk. These are also used extensively in societies where getting domestic help or nurses is relatively inexpensive or where people are unable to afford the other options.

Advancement in materials and manufacturing has resulted in significant improvements in these wheelchairs. These have led to wheelchairs that are lightweight and stronger. Improved seating and cushions, provision of head-stabilizing support, and seat belts are some of the useful options that allow the user to be more comfortable. There are also options where hand pedals and brakes are provided to control the wheelchair.

2.3.2 Motorized (Electric-Powered) Wheelchair

2.3.2.1 System Description

Improved power electronics systems started the motorization of wheelchairs; although earlier attempts simply added motors and batteries to manual wheelchairs, these have evolved greatly since then. While the majority of the motorized wheelchairs are provided with four wheels on a chassis, some are also provided with additional wheels to improve stability. Today, motorized wheelchairs no longer have the back wheels as large as their manual counterparts and are designed to provide a low center of gravity, while supporting the relatively very heavy batteries and motors. These wheelchairs are generally fabricated of steel, although aluminium and carbon-fiber-based frames are also being made available. From the very basic chair, these have evolved and improved electronics provide adaptive cushioning and support to the user. Some of these are also provided with features such as sensor-based navigation and emergency calling.

Modern wheelchairs are provided with smart and easy-to-use controllers that can be used to maneuver these chairs. Some of the more recent ones are provided with multiple motors that allow the user to travel through rough terrain and over small obstacles, and are also provided with adaptive control mechanisms that adapt to changes in the posture of the users.

The typical weight of the powered wheelchairs ranges from 36 to 70 kg, and the span of the chassis is typically 1040 mm (long) and 530 mm (wide). These chairs are provided with motors having a range of power output from 100 to 320 W (at 24 V), and the batteries (typically sealed lead acid of 12 V with capacity from 40 to 60 Ah) are long life. Once charged, the batteries can provide more than five hours of continuous use (or more than 30 km) to the wheelchair navigation, after which these require the batteries to be recharged. The maximum speed of these wheelchairs is typically 8 km/h, although most users would use them at relatively slower speeds. These are manufactured by many companies around the world; some of the global leaders are Invacare, Sunrise Medical, GF Health Products, Pride Mobility, Permobil, Colours in Motion, Quickie, Millennium, and LifeCare. The cost of these ranges between US$1,000 and US$15,000, and this difference is based on the need for customization and special features, as well as the health insurance policies of the country.

The other option to the traditional motorized wheelchair are ones suitable for rougher terrain, and these can be considered to be the four-wheel-drive equivalent. This all-terrain wheelchair uses two batteries of 75 Ah and motors from 900 to 1800 W, and has battery life up to 24 km. These tend to be more expensive, around US$20,000.

2.3.2.2 User Requirements

Motorized wheelchairs can be used by people who are able to control the wheelchair without colliding with other people or obstacles. The wheelchairs that are currently available require the users to have sufficient control and strength in their upper limbs to control the joystick and sufficient visual capability to be able to see people, obstacles, and dangerous situations.

These wheelchairs are generally suitable for places that have quality walkways and footpaths, with suitable road-crossing pathways that are suitable for wheelchairs, and for buildings that are designed for wheelchair access. Most of these wheelchairs are not suitable for cities where the infrastructure does not support wheelchairs, or where the pathways are not made of suitable quality to allow these wheelchairs to move easily. Another requirement for the effective usage of these chairs is the need for low-level traffic density and for the automobile traffic to be disciplined.

2.3.2.3 User Benefits

Motorized wheelchairs have revolutionized the lives of millions of people, giving these people a new lease on life. These wheelchairs facilitate social inclusion for the user, and people with disabilities are able to enjoy similar lifestyles compared with other people. The users can go to restaurants, attend meetings, and even enjoy many social activities. However, these benefits are limited to the relatively wealthy societies and for people living in planned cities. The high cost of the equipment along with poor infrastructure makes the use of these wheelchairs limited in poorer societies.

2.3.3 Mobility Scooter

The world population is aging rapidly. Approximately 10.8 percent of the Brazilian population is over 60 years of age [4]. In Australia this number is bigger, 18.6 percent, and with the aging "Baby Boomers," this proportion is expected to increase by 6 percent by 2020 [5]. Age-associated reduction in muscle control and an increase in the variation in force of muscle contraction leading to injuries and falls among the elderly is widely accepted. To help these people live an active lifestyle, mobility scooters are available. These devices are suitable for people who are able to walk, but fatigue very quickly, and require assistance. Mobility scooters are powered scooters that have motors and rechargeable batteries. While most of these come with four wheels, some three-wheeled options are also on the market.

2.3.3.1 System Description

Mobility scooters are generally battery-powered scooters with one seat and a handle bar, similar to the conventional scooter, although petrol engines are also available on special order. Unlike the conventional scooter, it has four (or sometimes three) wheels. These are designed for the elderly, provided with a shopping basket, and expected to be used in suburban areas or in retirement villages. While there are many brands and models, the major differences are in the aesthetics and in features such as the seat.

Compared with typical wheelchairs, mobility scooters are faster and can travel at a maximum speed of about 15 km/h, although devices capable of 60+ km/h have been reported (although would not be legal).

2.3.3.2 User Requirements

Mobility scooters are not considered to be vehicles but assistive technologies, and thus, in general, a driver's license is not required. Most people, even those who have never driven, are easily able to learn and use the mobility scooters. However, for the safety of the user and other people, some basic safeguards are that the person should be mentally alert and have upper limb control and strength to maneuver the scooter handle-bars.

Mobility scooters are suitable for places such as suburbs, shopping centers, and such places where there are quality walkways and footpaths, with suitable ramps to allow road crossings, and for buildings that are designed for wheelchair access. Effective usage of these scooters also requires low traffic density.

2.3.3.3 User Benefits and Future Development

Mobility scooters have given a new lease on life to the elderly and the infirm. For societies such as Australia and Brazil, where the population is rapidly aging, such equipment is very useful, because it allows the elderly to enjoy their independence and assists in their social inclusion. These devices are also very useful for reducing falls among the elderly.

The people who use mobility scooters often suffer from other difficulties such as arthritis, poor eyesight, and early fatigue. This results in their inability to use these devices for extended periods of time and also can result in accidents, especially when there are edges without edge-protective railings. Thus, there is a need to provide the mobility scooters with safety features such as edge detection, and for adaptive controllers that can reduce the impact of joint stiffness and muscle fatigue on the user's ability to maneuver the scooter.

References

[1] Reateam. http://reateam.com.br/detalhes-produto/avd-aluminio, accessed Jan 7, 2013.

[2] TopChair. http://www.topchair.fr/en/index_en.php, accessed Jan 7, 2013.

[3] Dezeen. http://www.dezeen.com/2012/09/05/paralympic-design-3d-printed-seats-for-wheelchair-basketball, accessed Jan 7, 2013.

[4] IBGE. http://www.ibge.gov.br, accessed June 30, 2013.

[5] ABS 2009, Disability Australia. http://www.abs.gov.au/ausstats/abs @.nsf/mf/4446.0, accessed Dec 10, 2012.

3

Smart Wheelchairs

André Ferreira, Sandra Müller, Wanderley Celeste, Daniel Cavalieri, Alessandro Benevides, Patrick Filgueira, Paulo Amaral, Mário Sarcinelli-Filho, and Teodiano Freire Bastos-Filho
Universidade Federal do Espírito Santo, Brazil

Elisa Perez and Carlos Soria
Universidad Nacional de San Juan, Argentina

CONTENTS

3.1 Introduction

Powered wheelchairs have overcome the limitations of millions of humans, and these are now visible in all major cities around the world. These have partially solved the mobility problems of people who are unable to walk. Typically, these are controlled by the user with the help of a joystick and require the user to manipulate the joystick, and thus it is necessary for the user to have sufficient control of his/her hand. It is also important for the users of these chairs to have reasonable eyesight to identify obstacles and people in the vicinity, and have a reasonable ability to react to situations in the proximity of the wheelchair. While the powered wheelchairs have been helpful to millions of people, there are many people who are unable to use these chairs due to the above reasons.

Smart wheelchairs have been under development since the beginning of the 1980s. The aim of these chairs is to overcome some of the limitations of powered wheelchairs and make these suitable for people who are unable to manipulate the joystick. Research and development in this area has been taking place in many countries and research laboratories.

In general, the basic principle of smart wheelchairs has been to obtain commands from the user from modalities other than the joystick, making these suitable for people who have or limited control of their hands. Some recent developments have been toward making these chairs semiautonomous and provide additional features that are suitable for users who are unable to manage their own mobility due to loss of memory, eyesight, or other complications. Other developments also include dynamic balancing to assist people who are unable to manage their balance on the chair. These are commonly referred to as robotic wheelchairs.

To extend the capabilities of the wheelchairs so that they are usable by those who are unable to control them using a joystick, research began in the early 1980s in several different countries. Some options are possible for controlling the wheelchair by a person who lacks hand control or sufficient strength.

Wheelchairs that provide navigation tools for helping a person navigate the wheelchair in between obstacles, especially for a person with reduced vision or reaction capabilities, have also been developed. Some of the navigation assistance techniques that help the users to make their mobility collision-free travel include identifying obstacles using ultrasound, image analysis, or GPS, or by using predefined pathways. There are also robotic wheelchairs that are programmed for autonomously transporting the user between predefined locations, such as described below [1]–[5].

3.2 Descriptions of Smart Wheelchairs

Smart wheelchairs consist of support for people who are unable to use the joystick by providing them with alternate wheelchair control options. These may also be provided with technology to assist the user in navigation or require safety features to prevent collisions. Some of these are also equipped for managing on uneven paths and even on stairs. Some of these features are described below.

3.2.1 Alternate Wheelchair Control Options

There have been a number of attempts to develop wheelchair controls that do not require the user to manipulate the joystick. Some of the options are (i) digital tablet, (ii) eye blinks, (iii) eye-gaze movements, (iv) head or face movements, (v) blowing and sucking (also named "sip and puff switch"), (vi) brain waves recorded from the surface, (vii) surface recording muscle electrical activity, and (viii) speech operated using a microphone. The complexity of these different options is highly varying. While the digital tablet is an extension of commercially available devices, the brain-wave-controlled devices are required to be developed and trained for an individual.

3.2.2 Digital Tablet and Touch-Screen Control

Digital tablet and touch screens are touch sensitive and allow the user to slide a finger on a flat tablet. They are similar to the computer mouse pad, and the user is able to give the commands for controlling the wheelchair using this. Such control has the advantage that it is inexpensive and can easily replace the joystick with minimal alterations to the wheelchair controller.

Touch screens allow the user to slide a finger in any direction, and this is commonly used in laptops and smartphones. Touch screens have also been used to control and direct a smart wheelchair. The Victoria, of Aachen University (2004), was a wheelchair equipped with two computers and a touch screen, cameras, and a manipulator. The user could control the wheelchair by sliding a finger over the touch screen. The system allows the user to manipulate the chair and additional equipment allows the user to grasp an object in close proximity. The grasped object could be placed on the wheelchair table, kept in the gripper, or held near the face of the user.

3.2.3 Eye-Blink or Eye-Gaze Tracking Controller

An option to give a command for people who may not have suitable strength or control of their hands is the use of their eyes. There are two options that are available: use of eye blinks or the use of eye gaze. Eye blinks allow the user to give simple commands using a series of blinks, and the most convenient method for identifying the blink is the use of eye muscle activity, recorded using surface electrodes located on the forehead. Eye-blink control has the advantage of simplicity in the hardware. However, involuntary eye blinks can lead to noise and, with binary commands, results in a very low bit rate, making it suitable for a very simple command structure.

An alternate is the use of an eye-tracking interface with a set of icons. The advantage of the eye-gaze-based control of wheelchair direction is that it is very natural to the user, who has to gaze in the direction of the desired movement. It was incorporated in the Wheelesley (1995) of MIT. This wheelchair used icons on a panel onboard to choose among different high-level movement commands, such as forward, left, right, stop, or drive backwards, while the direction command was obtained from eye tracking. The WASTON Project of NAIST (Japan, 2001) was a wheelchair with machine vision to interpret the user's gaze for directing the wheelchair.

3.2.4 Speech-Based Controller

Speech-based commands are very natural because of their richness and the ability for all people to communicate in their language. Another advantage is that it requires minimal hardware, only requiring a microphone and minimal training for the user. The wheelchair developed for the TAO Project (1996) of Applied AI Systems Inc. had a microphone, a keypad, and a joystick for onboard control interfaces. The user gave auditory commands such as stop, turn left, turn right, and drive. However, one difficulty of all audio-based systems is that these are limited to use where the ambient noise level is low.

The RobChair (1998) of the University of Coimbra was a wheelchair equipped with five wheels, and could be operated by voice, keyboard, and/or by an analog joystick. The Voice-cum-Auto Steer Wheelchair of CEERI (India, 1999) was voice commanded, used a small dictionary, and was suitable for being commanded to a prespecified given destination. This reduced the impact of noise on the ability of the system to identify user commands.

The FRIEND (Functional Robot arm with user-friendly Interface for Disabled people) of the University of Bremen (2001) had two parts: a wheelchair and a 6-degree-of-freedom robot arm. Both devices were controlled by a speech-recognition system.

3.2.5 Muscle Activity Control

People who have intact muscles, but the muscles are very weak or fatigue very quickly, are unable to move the joystick effectively. A system that recognizes the muscle activity of the user to identify the command issued is very natural to the user, and it overcomes the limitation due to fatigue or weakness. Electrical activity of the muscle can be recorded from the surface in the proximity of the muscle and this is referred to as surface electromyogram (sEMG). The HaWCos of the University of Siegen (2002) was a wheelchair that used muscle contractions as input signals. The DREAM-3 of Tottori University (2004) was a wheelchair that had five action patterns: follow the left wall, follow the right wall, turn left, turn right, and drive forward. The SWCS (Smart Wheelchair

Component System) of the University of Pittsburgh (2004) navigated using information from ultrasonic sensors, infrared, and bump sensors.

3.2.6 Head Movement

By tilting the head, a user can give directional commands to the wheelchair. This is suitable for people who have limited options, but one of the biggest drawbacks of such a system is that the users are unable to use it for extended periods of time at any given time. One example of the use of head movement for smart wheelchair control is the Intelligent Wheelchair System of Osaka University (1998), which had two cameras, one facing toward the user and the other facing forward. Users provided input to the system with head gestures, interpreted by the inward-facing camera.

3.2.7 Hybrid Control Options

Different wheelchair users have highly varying sets of capabilities and limitations, and to make a smart wheelchair that is suitable for a large number of people, a controller that allows the user to give commands using different inputs is a good option. The SIAMO project at the University of Alcala (1999) was used as a test bed for various input methods (voice, face/head gestures, EOG) for the wheelchair.

The SPAM (Smart Power Assistance Module) of the University of Pittsburgh (2005) used torque sensors to measure the manual forces applied and dynamically altered the required torque to reduce the risk of fatigue.

The robotic wheelchair of UFES/Brazil provides the flexibility for users to choose different modalities to command the wheelchair, using their eye blinks, eye movements, head movements, blow and suck (on a straw), and brain signals recorded using surface-mounted electrodes.

3.2.8 Smart Wheelchairs: Obstacle Detection

Powered wheelchairs are now fast and powerful, and can, like other mobility machines, cause injuries if they run into an obstacle. These require careful control to ensure that the user and other people in his/her proximity are safe. However, a number of users of such equipment have reduced vision, are slow to react, and may also have reduced control. This increases the chances of collisions, so there is the need for proximity sensing. Another limitation with the common powered wheelchair is that it is limited to use on flat terrain and cannot go over rough surfaces or on steps.

There are number of options for detecting obstacles, such as the use of laser, ultrasound or infrared sensors, or tactile and proximity sensors. Video analysis is also an option for identifying the obstacles.

The pioneer in assistive navigation wheelchairs was the Smart-Alec project at Stanford University (1980). They used ultrasonic sensors to detect the user's position and prevent collisions. An extension of the Smart Alec was the Madarasz wheelchair (1986), developed at Arizona State University, which was equipped with ultrasonic sensors and able to navigate through corridors. Further improvements, using multiple sensors, can be excmplified by the NavChair of the University of Michigan (1993), which was built to avoid obstacles, follow walls, and travel safely in cluttered environments using ultrasound sensors. Tin Man I and Tin Man II, of KISS Institute for Practical Robotics, also employed ultrasound sensors for obstacle avoidance and extended the chair's capabilities to sense the presence of a table for docking purposes. The Wheelesley (1995) of MIT was a wheelchair equipped with infrared proximity sensors and ultrasonic range sensors.

The wheelchair of the University of Pennsylvania (1994) was equipped with two legs in addition to the four regular wheels; the legs enabled the wheelchair to climb stairs and move through rough terrain. The Smart Wheelchair (1995) of the University of Edinburgh had bump sensors to sense low-level obstacles and had a line-following algorithm for driving through narrow regions such as doorways and corridors between rooms. The Orpheus (1996) of the University of Athens was a wheelchair equipped with 15 ultrasonic sensors for localization and obstacle avoidance, and had four basic actions: move straight, turn left, turn right, and reverse.

The wheelchair developed in the TAO Project (1996) of Applied AI Systems Inc. had functions for collision avoidance, driving in narrow corridors, and driving through narrow doorways, using two color cameras to identify colored landmarks.

The Rhombus (Reconfigurable Holonomic Omnidirectional Mobile Bed with Unified Seating) of MIT (1997) was a wheelchair with omnidirectional drive and could be reconfigured into a bed. The RobChair (1998) of the University of Coimbra was equipped with 12 infrared sensors, four ultrasonic sensors, and one tactile sensor located on the front bumper. The Hephaestus of TRACLabs (1999) was also equipped with 16 ultrasonic sensors, and these were configured to detect obstacles of different sizes.

The INRO (Intelligenter Rollstuhl) of the University of Applied Sciences Ravensburg-Weingarten (1998) was made with the main objective to support users with disabilities in navigation and for obstacle detection.

3.2.9 Autonomous Navigation and Control

Many wheelchair users are unable to give motion commands that can be identified accurately by the wheelchair controller. In some cases, this may happen for a short duration, while for others, this may be a regular condition. For such people, there is a need for wheelchairs to have some level of autonomy that can assist the user to define and reach the destination. Some examples of the wheelchairs that have been developed over the past 20 years are provided in Section 3.3.

3.3 Autonomous Wheelchairs over 20 Years

The Smart Wheelchair of the University of Plymouth (1998) and also of the University of Hong Kong (2002) used a controller based on neural networks to trace predefined paths autonomously within an art gallery.

The Luoson III of National Chung Cheng University (1999) was equipped with a force reflection joystick, video camera, ultrasonic sensors, digital compass, gyroscope, and microphone. It had three operating modes: direct control, assistive control, and autonomous control. In the autonomous control mode, it was designed for a restricted area, the details of which were programmed into the wheelchair controller.

The OMNI (Office wheelchair with high Maneuverability and Navigational Intelligence) of the University of Hagen (1999) had omnidirectional steering and was equipped with ultrasonic sensors and an infrared detector for real-time obstacle avoidance and back tracing. The wheelchair controller recorded the commanded path in the memory, and this was to assist the user of the wheelchair to return to the original location without effort.

The VAHM (French acronym for autoVehicule Autonome pour Handicape Moteurnomous) of the University of Metz (1993, 2001) used a grid-based method for navigation. The SmartChair of the University of Pennsylvania (2002) was equipped with wheel encoders, an omnidirectional camera, infrared sensors, a laser range finder, and an interaction camera, and had six behaviors (control modes): hallway navigation, three-point turn (reversing and turning), obstacle avoidance, navigation through a doorway, turn while avoiding an obstacle, and direction to a specific goal.

The SIRIUS of the University of Seville (2002) was a wheelchair that could be teleoperated, run autonomously, or be manually controlled. The Collaborative Wheelchair Assistant of National University (Singapore, 2002) allowed users to travel according to predefined paths. The SPAM (Smart Power Assistance Module) of the University of Pittsburgh (2005) was a wheelchair that used information from different types of sensors (ultrasonic and infrared) for assistive navigation. The TAO Aicle of AIST (National Institute of Advanced Industrial Science and Technology of Japan, 2006) incorporated a laser range finder for mapping the pathway, GPS to identify the location, compass to determine the direction, and radio frequency identification (RFID) for determining the location of predefined locations, and for locating itself.

The Rolland I (2001) of the University of Bremen and MAid (Mobility Aid for Elderly and Disabled People) of the University of Ulm (2001) were equipped with a large number of ultrasonic sensors and a laser range finder for obstacle avoidance and navigation, while Rolland III and Argyro's Wheelchairs of the Institute of Computer Science (Greece, 2002) were also equipped with omnidirectional cameras (used to find features in the environment). The WAD Project of the Centre National de la Recherche Scientifique (CNRS) (2002) was a wheelchair that could avoid obstacles through infrared sensors.

3.3.1 Markers and RFID for Navigation

When the wheelchair users are unable to provide commands that can be accurately interpreted by the wheelchair controller, floor markers and RFID-based systems can be used for helping the user travel between fixed locations, such as the television room and the bedroom. The advantage of these is that they are inexpensive and reliable, while the disadvantage of these is that they are only suitable for small areas where the paths can be predefined. Floor markers may be visual or magnetic, and RFID may also be used to identify the location of different objects and the wheelchair itself. The Tetranuta (1999) of the University of Seville was provided with a navigation system using landmarks painted on the floor and in the form of radio beacons. The Voice-cum-Auto Steer Wheelchair of CEERI (India, 1999) could autonomously travel to a given destination based on an internal map or by following tape paths on floor.

The robotic wheelchair of UFES/Brazil can be commanded by users in a supervised way or by a fully automatic, unsupervised onboard navigation system. The wheelchair can operate like an autoguided vehicle, following metallic tapes on the floor, or in an autonomous way. The system is provided with an easy-to-use and flexible graphical user interface running on a personal digital assistant (PDA), which allows users to choose destination commands to be sent to the robotic wheelchair, and an RFID system used to calibrate the wheelchair location during navigation.

3.3.2 Wheelchairs with General Purposes

The Walking Wheelchair of the University of Castilla–La Mancha (2006) was equipped with four wheels and four legs. The legs made it possible for the wheelchair to climb stairs. The HURI Project of Yonsei University (2002–2003) was a wheelchair with machine vision to identify facial gestures of the user. The WAD Project of Bochum University (2002) was a wheelchair that either navigated autonomously to a desired position or provided obstacle avoidance while the user navigated. Niigata University (2004) developed a wheelchair that used EOG signals to command a cursor to displace in four directions (up, down, left, and right) while one blink of the eye selected the icon. The University of Electrocommunication (Japan) and the University of Boston (USA), in 2004, developed a wheelchair that could be commanded by brain waves, using 13 electroencephalogram (EEG) electrodes. The University of Zaragoza (2009) developed a wheelchair commanded by voice, blowing, and brain waves.

The robotic wheelchair of Ecole Polytechnique Federale de Lausanne (EPFL, 2010) used camera, laser, and ultrasonic sensors, plus a collaborative controller, to help users safely drive the wheelchair, commanding it through eye movements. The ARTY (Assistive Robot Transport for Youngsters) of Imperial College London (2011) was a pediatric wheelchair equipped with ultrasonic and infrared sensors that could be commanded by children through head movements (captured by a gyroscope on a hat).

The IDIAP Research Institute (2011) developed a wheelchair that could be commanded by brain waves. Pohang University of Science and Technology (2012) used tongue movements to command a wheelchair, and the Federal University of Espirito Santo (UFES/Brazil, 2012) developed a robotic wheelchair with a unified platform based on eye blinks, eye movements, head movements, blowing and sucking, and brain waves to provide the user the choice of the most suitable modality to command the wheelchair. This wheelchair can operate in nonautonomous, autonomous, or semiautonomous ways.

3.3.3 Additional Possible Features for Robotic Wheelchairs

Many people with special needs who use smart wheelchairs are unable to communicate because they lack the motor skills for speech. Thus, incorporating devices that facilitate communication for people who are unable to speak is a natural progression. One example is the robotic wheelchair of UFES/Brazil, which has a communication system onboard that allows users to communicate with the people around them, as the wheelchair has two speakers onboard to emit an artificial voice according to the option of communication selected by the user.

3.4 Robotic Wheelchair of UFES/Brazil

A number of independent research groups and organizations have developed smart wheelchairs that have unique designs and features. However, the fundamentals of each of these are similar, with a number of commonalities in the basic design and the features. To best explain the design principle, the detailed design of one comprehensive smart wheelchair, the robotic wheelchair by UFES, is discussed below as an example.

The most significant difference between the usual powered wheelchairs and smart wheelchairs is the interface with which the user controls the chair. There are a number of different terminologies for these interfaces, such as human–computer interface (HCI) or man–machine interface (MMI). These are designed to obtain commands from the user and convert these to control signals for the wheelchair.

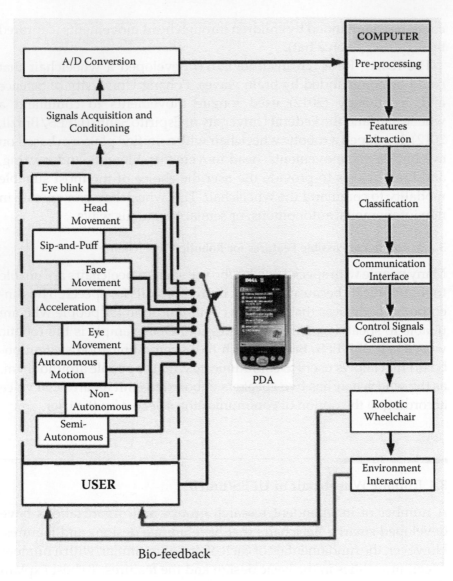

FIGURE 3.1
Structure of the developed human–machine interface.

Figure 3.1 shows the general structure of the human–machine interface (HMI) developed and installed onboard the robotic wheelchair of UFES/Brazil. This interface consists of an acquisition system that includes amplification, filtering, digitization, recording, and processing of different kinds of signals provided by the wheelchair user. The signals are recorded and classified in real time, sending the identified

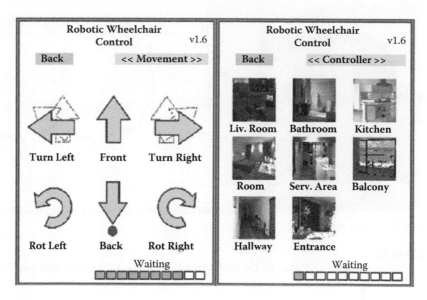

FIGURE 3.2
Different options of movement commands (arrows of movement or symbols representing places) presented on the PDA screen onboard the wheelchair. See color insert.

class to a PDA. This PDA is responsible for generating commands of movement to a computer onboard the wheelchair, to give feedback to the user, and to automatically perform a symbol scan. These symbols are associated with movements (arrows or destination places), as shown in Figure 3.2. Once a valid command is identified, a movement command actuates the wheelchair.

3.4.1 Commands by Eye Blinks

Surface electromyogram (sEMG) is the recording of the electrical activity generated at the surface near the muscle, when the muscle is contracting. sEMG signals recorded from above the frontal muscles are an indicator of the blink movement of the eyelids and thus used to identify eye blinks.

In the robotic wheelchair of UFES, this was recorded using a bioamplifier and then digitized and captured at a sampling rate of 1000 samples/second, using two electrodes located on frontal muscles, and one reference electrode placed on the right earlobe, as shown in Figure 3.3(a). One channel was used for the right eye muscle and the other one for the left eye muscle. A threshold was identified for the recording using pilot recording, and this was used to identify the beginning and

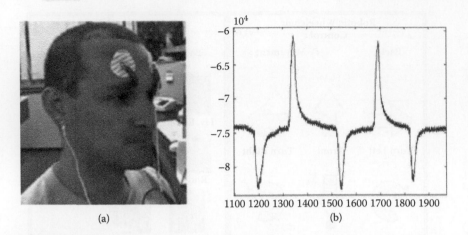

(a)   (b)

FIGURE 3.3
(a) sEMG acquisition (eye blinks). (b) Up: myoelectric signal due to blinks of the right eye; Down: blinks of the left eye.

the end of the eye-blink muscle activity. The duration of the blink was used to determine voluntary and involuntary eye blinks. The value of the threshold and the duration of the blink were determined by training a back-propagation neural network. The system that gave the best results was a neural network consisting of four hidden neurons and with the sEMG down-sampled by a factor of 20. The example of the recording is shown in Figure 3.3(b).

The resulting system was found to be reliable and accurate (99.6 percent of hit rate) but unsuitable for users with muscle spasms, excessive involuntary blinking, or loss of eye control.

3.4.2 Commands by Head or Face Movements

Two approaches have been provided for enabling the use of head movement to command the wheelchair. One approach uses an IMU (inertial measurement unit) attached to a cap (or other device attached to the head), called a gravitational acceleration system. The second approach is a video-based system that uses an onboard video camera mounted in front of the wheelchair, focusing on the user's face.

3.4.2.1 Head Movements Modality

The users can command the wheelchair by using their head or face movement. The robotic wheelchair of UFES has used an IMU, based on an accelerometer, attached to a cap or headband attached to the

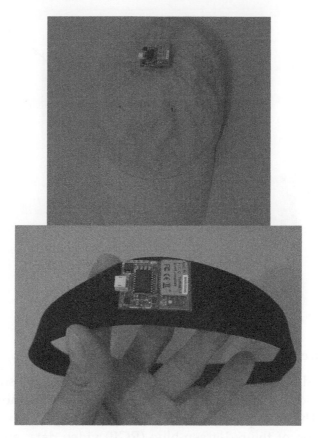

FIGURE 3.4
Inclination sensor based on IMU board attached to (a) cap; (b) headband.

head. The advantage of using head movement is the ease with which it can be incorporated and can be considered as a modified joystick, but which is operated by the head of the user and suitable for someone who does not have hand action control.

A two-axis IMU connected to the computer using Bluetooth and mounted on the cap of the user (Figure 3.4) was used to provide a voltage proportional to the head inclination. The user directs the wheelchair by tilting the head forward, to the right, or to the left, while tilting the head to the rear commands the wheelchair to stop.

The IMU-based smart wheelchair was found to be robust and reliable for people who had sufficient strength in their neck muscles. However, people who were unable to control their head tilt were unable to use this modality.

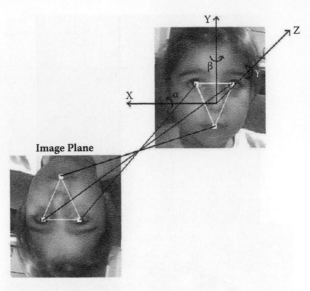

FIGURE 3.5
Facial features. See color insert.

3.4.2.2 Face Detection Modality

A standard lightweight fixed-focus video camera can also be used to obtain head/face movements by detecting the facial movements of the user. The first step in video data analysis is to perform a histogram equalization of the red-green-blue (RGB) video data, aiming at improving contrasts and overcoming lighting variations. The resulted data are transformed to YCbCr space, to detect the skin color. The image is segmented to identify the skin, using threshold values for Cb and Cr previously obtained from training trials. An elliptical region of interest (ROI) is generated and centered at the first image moment of the segmented image. An operation *AND* is executed between the ellipsis generated and the negative of the y component (Figure 3.5).

The next step is the identification of the centroids of the regions associated with both eyes and mouth. For that, data are filtered using a Kalman filter to improve the position estimate. Three noncollinear points in the camera coordinates define a triangle in the image plane, as shown in Figure 3.5. Changes in space points, due to head and face movements, are projected onto the image plane, thus changing the points in the image.

From the point projections on the image, different angles of the head movements can be obtained: rotation around the z axis, rotation around

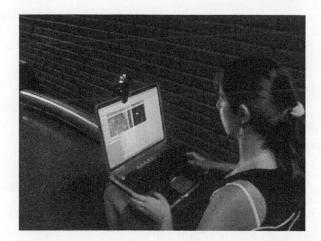

FIGURE 3.6
Robotic wheelchair commanded by head/face movements (captured by a video camera).

the y axis, and rotation around the x axis, respectively, by the following expressions:

$$\gamma = \tan^{-1}\left(\frac{yr - yl}{xr - xl}\right)$$

$$\beta = 2\tan^{-1}\left(\frac{a_1 \pm \sqrt{a_1^2 - f^2\left(a_1^2/a_0^2 - 1\right)}}{f\left(a_1/a_0 + 1\right)}\right)$$

$$\alpha = 2\tan^{-1}\left(\frac{c_1 \pm \sqrt{c_1^2 - f\left(c_1^2/c_0^2 - 1\right)}}{f\left(c_1/c_0 + 1\right)}\right)$$

Figure 3.6 shows the use of a video camera to capture images of the user's face, making it possible to command the wheelchair by head/face movements.

3.4.3 Commands by Blowing and Sucking

Blowing and sucking (also named sip and puff switch) can be used to command the wheelchair for users with the ability to blow and suck a straw. In this modality, a pressure sensor, installed into a straw, allows users either to choose icons of movement to be executed by the wheelchair or to choose the desired destination (Figure 3.7). This is

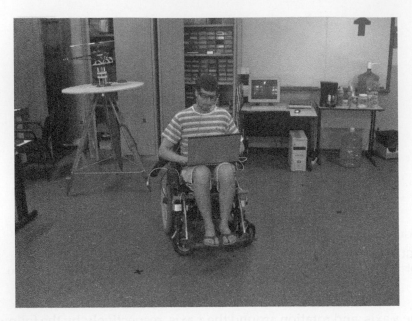

FIGURE 3.7
Robotic wheelchair commanded by blowing and sucking.

a simple, reliable, and inexpensive technique, and this modality was found to be robust but highly restrictive because it does not allow the user higher degrees of freedom for expression or command.

3.4.4 Commands by Eye Movements

Guiding the wheelchair using the direction of the eye gaze and eye movement has been found to be quite natural for people who are unable to use their hands. This can be achieved using electrical activity recorded from around the eye (called electrooculogram—EOG) or using video analysis. The robotic wheelchair of UFES has used the video technique (Figure 3.8). This requires a customized pair of glasses with a mounted and prefocused camera for detecting eye movements while a tablet-based computer displays a set of icons on the PDA screen. The user stares at the icon, and the higher gaze is recognized by the video analysis and used to control the wheelchair.

In this modality, the first step requires determining the ocular globe position for which some image-processing techniques are required for identification of the iris. A Hough Circular Random Transform and a Canny filter eliminate the influence of artifacts such as the eyebrow and

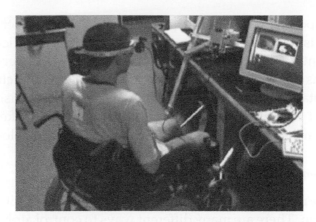

FIGURE 3.8
Robotic wheelchair commanded by eye movements.

eyelash. The next step requires the definition of the ROI around the eye to allow tracking of the eye movements. One of the limitations of the visual analysis method is the sensitivity to illumination variations and to camera noise. To overcome this, a Kalman filter was incorporated to denoise the image.

This system is robust and allows people with a high level of spinal cord injury to maneuver the wheelchair. However, there are people who cannot move the eyes, such as people at the final stage of ALS (also called Lou Gehrig's disease), a situation named "locked-in." For such people, another modality of wheelchair command, based on brain waves, is discussed in the next section.

3.4.5 Commands by Brain Waves

The electrical activity associated with the brain can be recorded using electrodes located on the surface of the scalp and is called the electroencephalogram (EEG). This recording can be used by the user to control the wheelchair or other such devices, and such a system is referred to as the brain–computer interface (BCI). BCI can be controlled by an action or the thought of the user, and people who may not have access to any other modality can use BCI.

EEG is the tracking of electrical activity that corresponds to very complex neural activity and is a sum of a large number of neurons.

It is nonspecific, the signal magnitude is only a few microvolts, and there tends to be large background noise, making it difficult to accurately identify the thought command of the user. A number of different paradigms have been developed to identify the brain activity of the user to obtain commands for controlling the wheelchair using the BCI. The use of mental tasks, motor imagery, and visual evoked potential are three major techniques. Each of these is described below.

3.4.5.1 Mental Tasks

One of the paradigms to command the wheelchair is by altering the alpha rhythm. There are many different ways to control alpha activity in the brain, which includes the use of emotions or by using visual excitation and relaxation. One easy option is based on visual excitation (eyes should be kept open) and relaxation (eyes closed) [1]. To detect this, a pair of electrodes was placed on the occipital cortex (visual region), position O1 and O2, according to the International 10-20 Standard of Electrode Placement, and a reference electrode was placed on the right earlobe.

Figure 3.9 shows the electrode location on the occipital cortex and the brain signals generated when the wheelchair user has visual excitation (suppression of alpha rhythm) or visual relaxation (activation of alpha rhythm). This is called Event-Related Synchronization (ERS), and the decrease of the EEG power is called Event-Related Desynchronization (ERD).

To identify the two alpha activity conditions, the signal variance (VAR) was evaluated. This has the advantage of self-normalizing the magnitude of the signal. To overcome the noise issues, the signal was classified using two thresholds (higher and lower), with the region in between the two thresholds being the dead zone (Figure 3.10). This method reduces the number of false positives, although it would increase the number of unknowns. This is required to prevent any accidental command. Figure 3.11 shows the robotic wheelchair commanded by mental tasks.

3.4.5.2 Using Motor Imagery and Word Generation

EEG has been shown to correlate with imagination of the movement, and this is called motor imagery. Another option is to train the user to turn on a section of the brain based on the imagination of words.

When using motor imagery, the initial cognitive activity responsible for the intention of performing a motor task occurs in the brain cortex, over the frontal, prefrontal, and parietal lobes. This then propagates to the striatum and the motor loop at the base of the brain, and reaches the motor cortex through the thalamus. The change in the EEG has opposite laterality to the imagined action [2]. The change in the activity can be observed from electrodes over the motor cortex, the frontal lobe, and the parietal lobe [3].

When using the mental task of thinking of words such as the same first character, the correspondent pattern can be detected in the language-processing section of the brain (Broca's area). This can be captured by electrodes placed on the left hemisphere of the frontal and parietal lobes.

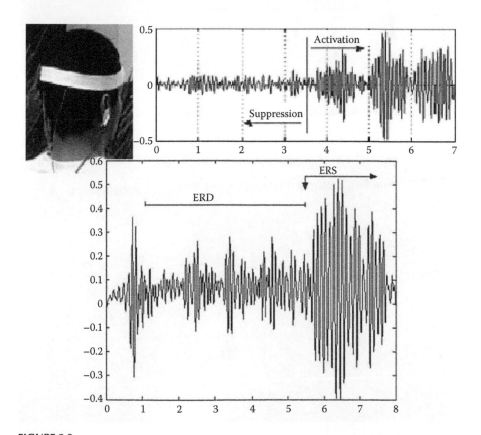

FIGURE 3.9
EEG acquisition on the occipital region, showing different energies of the EEG signal, due to (a) visual excitation (suppression of alpha rhythm) and visual relaxation (activation of alpha rhythm); (b) equivalent ERD/ERS patterns.

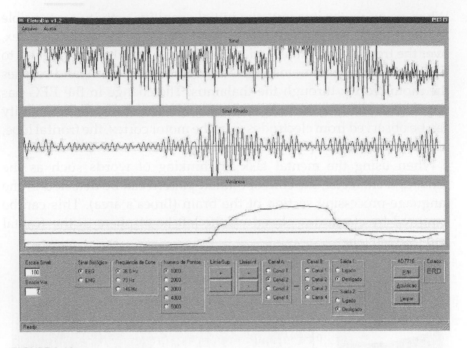

FIGURE 3.10
EEG signal with two thresholds used to get the right commands.

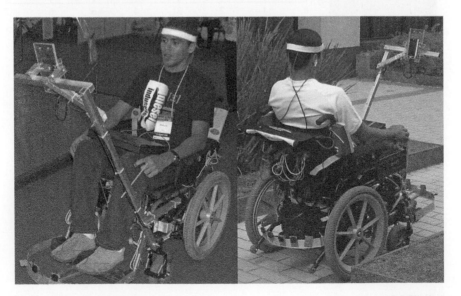

FIGURE 3.11
Robotic wheelchair commanded by mental tasks. See color insert.

The robotic wheelchair has considered the EEG corresponding to the user to imagine three options: movement of the right hand, of the left hand, and words beginning with the same letter. Power Spectral Density (PSD) of EEG using a moving window was classified using Linear Discriminant Analysis (LDA) and then measured using correlation analysis. The results of this technique reach a hit rate of up to 94.9 percent, with the user having high specificity.

3.4.5.3 Using Visual Evoked Potential

Another paradigm to command the wheelchair is using Steady State Visual Evoked Potential (SSVEP). The user has to gaze at the icon or direction arrow, which gives visual flickering stimulation, and the target of the gaze is identified because the frequency of this flickering stimulus is present in the EEG signal. In contrast with other BCIs, an SSVEP-BCI requires no user training or calibration and achieves a high information transfer rate (ITR) [4]. Also, this kind of BCI is easy to operate and configure, and is less susceptible to artifacts produced by eye blinks and eye movements because the EEG signal, recorded in the occipital area, is far from the source of such artifacts [5]. The robotic wheelchair of UFES uses four black/white checkerboard stripes flickering at 5.6 repetition per seconds–rps (top), 6.4 rps (right), 6.9 rps (bottom), and 8.0 rps (left), shown in Figure 3.12 and Figure 3.13. In this modality, brain waves are temporally and spatially filtered and then features are extracted by a statistical test called the Spectral F-Test (SFT). The results are used to identify the critical value and classified using a decision-tree-based classifier.

3.4.6 Communication System

The multimodal interface installed onboard the robotic wheelchair can be used for communication. The interface provides flexibility to choose different modalities for communication by people with different levels of disabilities. Users can use the interface through eye blinks, eye movements, head movements, by blowing or sucking a straw, and through brain signals. The PDA onboard displays different communication options, and gives visual feedback to the user (Figure 3.14). The communication and command options include icons that

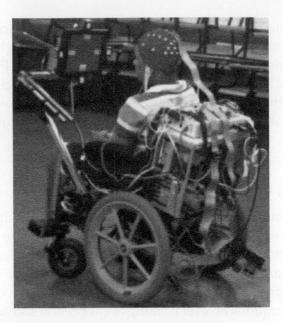

FIGURE 3.12
Robotic wheelchair commanded by SSVEP, according to the stripe (top, bottom, left, and right) gazed on by the user.

represent feelings or wishes, and letters to make sentences. A text-to-audio converter onboard the wheelchair is also provided to facilitate communication for the user. This interface can be used by people with poor language skills and also extended to other languages.

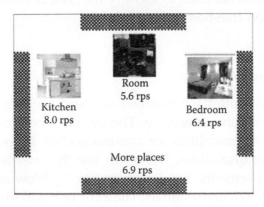

FIGURE 3.13
Visual stimuli used to choose destination places.

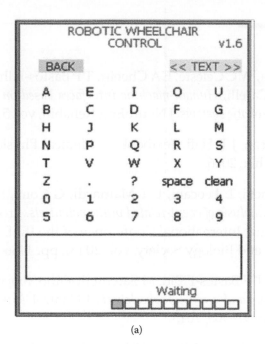

(a)

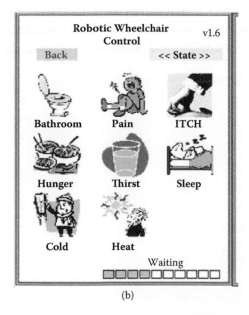

(b)

FIGURE 3.14

Options for communication: (a) letter to make sentences; (b) icons representing feelings or wishes. See color insert for (b).

References

[1] A Ferreira, W C Celeste, F A Cheein, T F Bastos-Filho, M Sarcinelli-Filho, R Carelli, *Human-machine interfaces based on EMG and EEG applied to robotic systems*. J NeuroEng Rehabili, vol. 5, pp. 1–15, 2008.

[2] A C Guyton, J E Hall, Textbook of Medical Physiology, 11th ed., Philadelphia, 2006.

[3] A M Bianchi, L Leocani, L T Mainardi, G Comi, S Cerutti, *Time-frequency analysis of event-related brain potentials*. Proceedings of the 20th Annual International Conference of the IEEE Engineering in Medicine and Biology Society, vol. 20 (3), pp. 1486–1489, 1998.

[4] S Muller, T F Bastos-Filho, M Sarcinelli-Filho, *Proposal of a SSVEP-BCI to command a robotic wheelchair*. J Control Autom Electr Syst, vol. 24, pp. 97–105, 2013.

[5] T L Mandel, T Laue, T Rofer, A Graser, B Krieg-Bruckner, *Navigating a smart wheelchair with a brain-computer interface interpreting steady-state visual evoked potentials*. Proceedings of IEEE/RSJ International Conference on Intelligent Robots and Systems, pp. 1118–1125, 2009.

4

Navigation System for UFES's Robotic Wheelchair

Fernando Cheein
Universidad Técnica Federico Santa María, Chile

Celso De La Cruz, Edgard Guimarães, and Teodiano Freire Bastos-Filho
Universidade Federal do Espírito Santo, Brazil

Ricardo Carelli
Universidad Nacional de San Juan, Argentina

CONTENTS

4.1 Introduction

The robotic wheelchair of UFES/Brazil provides an autoguided option to the user for indoor environment navigation, focused on autonomously solving complex maneuvers that would require too much effort from the user, especially for highly dependent ones. Additionally, the autonomous driving option of the robotic wheelchair can also be used when the user wants to reach a given location within the environment in a short time. Thus, the main aim of this mode is to minimize both the user's effort and a collision risk. The way the autonomous navigation mode is implemented on the navigation system of the wheelchair was previously shown in Figure 3.1.

In an autonomous navigation mode, the wheelchair and its user are no longer considered as a sole system. Instead, other actors play important roles in the navigation mode. Figure 4.1 shows this new scenario. Briefly,

- **Environment:** In the autonomous navigation mode, it is necessary to consider the environment during the driving of the robotic wheelchair, since the environment determines the

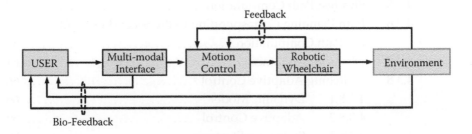

FIGURE 4.1
General architecture of the multimodal interface presented in Figure 3.1 with the autonomous navigation approach.

path-planning or trajectory-planning tasks, which are related to the wheelchair's motion controller and the user's own decisions. Thus, it is not the same to plan motion in a dynamic environment (e.g., other people moving around the wheelchair) as it is in a static one. The crucial role of the environment in the autonomous navigation mode is depicted in two examples in this chapter: the crossing-a-door problem (which is not trivial if the user does not have the capabilities for refining maneuvering of the wheelchair) and the turning-back problem. Thus, the environment acts as a constraining factor in the navigational system of the wheelchair.

- **Control system:** Although the motion control of the wheelchair is a well-known problem and several solutions have been published in the scientific literature [1] [2], the fact that the control has to include environment information is still an open issue. Furthermore, the control system should include the user's own preferences because comfort is an issue that the designer must take into account. For example, if the motion control causes centrifugal forces to be too high, the user's confidence regarding the device might be compromised. Thus, a solution from the control systems field should also consider the user as a crucial variable in the design.

- **Feedback:** This stage needs special mention. Despite the fact that biofeedback is mandatory for every human–machine interface, in autonomous systems the quality of the feedback determines the success or failure of the autonomous navigation per se. For example, if the wheelchair is following a predefined path, the knowledge of the wheelchair's location within the environment is necessary for control actions. A bad positioning system could lead to risky maneuvers or collisions with the environment, compromising the user's safety. Additionally, the localization system and the knowledge of the surrounding environment can be used to expand the wheelchair's reachable space, from indoors to outdoors, thus augmenting the user's motion capabilities [3]. These topics are covered in the following sections.

As can be seen in Figure 4.1, the user of the robotic wheelchair receives biofeedback from the environment (i.e., the user learns from the environment and uses such information for driving the wheelchair), from the wheelchair per se (i.e., the user learns about the behavior of the wheelchair and how to use it), and from the interface [3] [4] [5]. On the other hand, the autonomous navigation approach needs feedback from the environment (it uses the environment information for motion planning) and from the robotic wheelchair (e.g., dead-reckoning sensors are able to provide position estimation).

4.2 Environment Information

As previously stated, the environment plays the most important role in the autonomous navigation mode of the robotic wheelchair. Therefore, in this chapter, two approaches are shown in which the environment is interpreted in different ways. The first approach uses metallic tapes previously and strategically distributed all around a conservative environment (i.e., structured and adequate for wheelchair navigation). The second approach considers a SLAM (Simultaneous Localization and Mapping) algorithm implemented on the wheelchair for navigation, control, and recognition of new environments. Both approaches are studied in the following sections.

4.2.1 Metallic Tapes–Based Environment Disposition

This specific approach consists of placing Y-shaped metallic tapes on the floor of a structured environment. Such metallic tapes can be used for navigation within the environment or for precise maneuvering. Figure 4.2 shows a schematic of the metallic tapes disposition.

Although the metallic tapes have been used in this application for solving the crossing-a-door problem, they can be also used for navigation [4]. Thus, each Y-shaped metallic tape can be considered as a node, and a topological map of the environment can be obtained and used for navigational purposes. Nevertheless, in places where no metallic tapes are available—short dashed lines in Figure 4.2—the user should drive the wheelchair using a different mode. More about this technique is explained later herein.

It is worth mentioning that the wheelchair and the environment need adaptation in order to efficiently drive following the mentioned

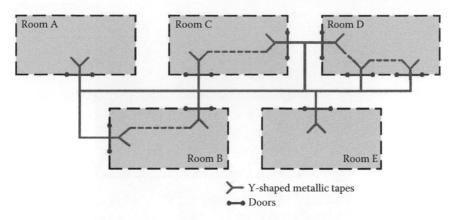

FIGURE 4.2
Example of Y-shaped metallic tapes placement.

metallic tapes. Thus,

- Magnetic sensors are installed on the wheelchair which detect the metallic tracks.
- In the autoguided option, the pathway for the wheelchair along the metallic tapes, from the current location to the desired destination, is determined by the wheelchair's onboard computer.
- RFID (Radio Frequency Identification) tags are also installed in suitable locations, such as doors, to calibrate dead reckoning.
- The system also provides acoustic feedback to the user for location awareness.

Figure 4.3 shows details of the magnetic sensors and the RFID reader installed onboard the wheelchair.

The navigation system implemented in this modality is limited by the number of possible destinations [4], which are offered to the user through the PDA. For example, room A can be the living room of the user's house, and once a destination is chosen, the system will plan the appropriate path following the metallic tapes until the wheelchair has reached the desired destination point. The localization of the robotic wheelchair within the environment is mainly based on dead reckoning with the RFID system implemented on it. In particular, the RFID system allows the wheelchair to recognize that it has reached the desired room.

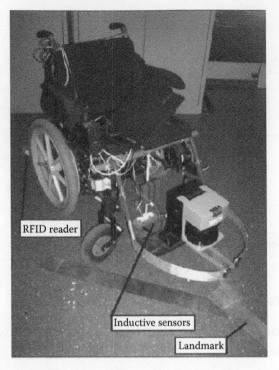

FIGURE 4.3
Details of the inductive sensors and their location on the robotic wheelchair, RFID reader, landmark, metallic tracks, and a laser sensor mounted at the wheelchair's footrest.

4.2.2 SLAM-Based Environment Learning

The SLAM (Simultaneous Localization and Mapping) algorithm concurrently (and recursively) estimates both the position of the vehicle and the surrounding environment. In order to do so, the SLAM algorithm requires the following:

- A sensor to acquire information from the environment. Several sensors can be used for this purpose, such as range sensors (laser and ultrasonic) and vision systems (TOF—time of flight—cameras; monocular, binocular, and trinocular vision systems; as well as stereo vision). In addition, recently 3D vision systems such as the Kinect (built by Microsoft) are being used in assistive vehicles [6] [7].

- A motion model associated with the sensor. This is a common mistake in SLAM algorithms: The designer associates the

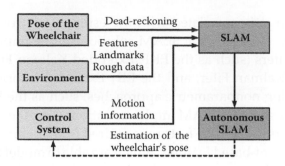

FIGURE 4.4
SLAM and Autonomous SLAM.

kinematic model of the vehicle with the estimation process. However, it is the motion of the sensor on the vehicle that matters. Thus, for example, the vehicle might have Ackermann constraints and yet the sensor's motion is the unicycle type [8].

- An environment information model. The latter seeks to answer the following question: Which features from the environment are useful for mapping? Several answers apply to this question: from line segments associated to walls in indoors environments, to point-based features associated with corners or with trees in outdoors environments [9] [10], to rough data acquired by, e.g., a 3D LiDAR system. It is important not to forget that the information extracted from the environment is intrinsically related to the nature of the environment and the sensor [10]. Thus, a SLAM algorithm designed for indoors might not work properly outdoors due to sensor constraints and the absence of features. For example, a tree-based SLAM algorithm (as the one shown in [9]) will certainly not work indoors.

Figure 4.4 shows a general description of the SLAM algorithm. It uses the environment information, the dead-reckoning information provided by the wheelchair, and the motion control information to estimate the vehicle's position within the environment and to map such an environment at the same time. In addition, if the position estimation is used by the control system, then the SLAM algorithm is named *autonomous SLAM* [11].

A parametric representation of the SLAM algorithm is basically composed of two elements: the SLAM system state and the SLAM covariance matrix associated with the estimation error of the vector system state. A parametric SLAM solution can be implemented in a variety of filters (such as the EKF, Extended Kalman Filter; the UKF, Unscented Kalman Fiter; and the EIF, Extended Information Filter), and also using nonparametric approaches, such as the Particle Filter. Equation 4.1 shows a SLAM implementation using the EIF, presented by the authors in [12]. The features acquired from the environment correspond to point-based features, which are able to model both trees and corners from the environment, thus being able to perform a consistent indoors and outdoors SLAM algorithm.

$$
\begin{cases}
\mu_{t-1} = \Upsilon_{t-1}^{-1}\xi_{t-1} \\
\bar{\Upsilon}_t = (G_t\Upsilon_{t-1}^{-1}G_t^T + Q_t)^{-1} \\
\bar{\xi}_t = \bar{\Upsilon}_t g(u_t, \mu_{t-1}) \\
\bar{\mu}_t = g(u_t, \mu_{t-1}) \\
\Upsilon_t = \bar{\Upsilon}_t + H_t^T R_t^{-1} H_t \\
\xi_t = \bar{\xi}_t + H_t^T R_t^{-1}[z_t - h(\bar{\mu}_t) + H_t\bar{\mu}_t]
\end{cases}
\tag{4.1}
$$

where μ is the system state vector (which contains the position of the vehicle and the location of the extracted features from the environment); ξ and Υ, the information matrix, are the parameters of the EIF. It is to be noted that ξ and μ are of the same dimension, and Υ has the same dimension as the covariance matrix associated with μ ($\Upsilon^{-1} = \Omega$, the covariance matrix of the SLAM at the system state μ). Additionally, G is the Jacobian matrix of the vehicle's motion model, and Q its associated covariance matrix; u is the control command input; H is the Jacobian matrix of the features' mathematical model, and R is the covariance matrix of the sensor; z is the feature acquired from the environment, and $\bar{\xi}$ and $\bar{\Upsilon}$ are the predicted parameters of the EIF; see [12] for further details.

4.2.3 SLAM vs. Metallic Tapes

Both the SLAM algorithm and the metallic tapes approaches present advantages and drawbacks that have to be taken into account before implementing an autoguided robotic wheelchair. Table 4.1 shows a comparison between both approaches.

TABLE 4.1

Pros and Cons of the SLAM and the Metallic Tapes Approaches

Metallic Tapes	SLAM
The tapes have to be previously placed in the environment, increasing the costs of the system and narrowing the reachable workspace of the robotic wheelchair	The exteroceptive sensor of the wheelchair is able to map the surrounding environment. However, the wheelchair should navigate the environment at least once in order to obtain a map of it
The navigation environment is restricted by the tapes' disposition on the floor, and the wheelchair's maneuvering is constrained to such disposition	The SLAM algorithm provides information that a path-planning or a path-tracking technique can use in order to enhance the navigation procedure
The metallic tapes–based navigation system requires a magnetic sensor. Such a sensor is very unlikely to show inconsistences in the readings since floors are not usually metallic. Therefore, the control can be very refined and stable	SLAM algorithms are always sensitive to inconsistences in the estimation procedure. They are strongly dependent on the type of sensor used and thus they depend on the nature of the environment. If the SLAM algorithm does not detect any useful features from the environment, then it might diverge in time. This situation represents a risk to the user since position estimation is no longer reliable
Metallic tapes approach is a hardware-based solution	The SLAM algorithm is a software-based solution

4.2.4 Motion Control and Feedback

Whether the wheelchair's navigation system is based on metallic tapes or SLAM information, the wheelchair per se needs a control strategy in order to ensure that it performs the appropriate motion to achieve the user's request. However, the control strategy is strongly related to the localization system implemented. Thus, readings from dead reckoning are quite different from SLAM position estimations of the wheelchair: Although both estimate the wheelchair's position, only odometry—i.e., dead reckoning—gives a position estimation that does not violate the nonholonomic constraints of the vehicle. The following presents how the control strategy and the entire navigational system of the wheelchair are prepared for both metallic tapes and SLAM-based approaches.

4.3 Metallic Tapes–Based Navigation

For the wheelchair navigation, structured environments such as the case of a typical house are considered. Every landmark installed is composed of a segment of metallic path and an RFID tag. These landmarks are placed in several locations, such as doorways, passageways, and target positions. Every segment of metallic path and RFID tag defines a node of a directed graph. This graph defines a topological map. The initial posture (position and orientation) and final posture of the wheelchair do not need to be over a segment of metallic path; nevertheless, these postures are also considered to be nodes of the graph. After generating the topological map, a shortest path from the initial to the final node on the graph is computed using the Dijkstra algorithm. A metric map is also used in the navigation system, and it is used in the path planning between pairs of landmarks. The localization procedure for this navigation system is based on encoders, inductive sensors, and an RFID reader. The odometry information is used for localization, which is corrected online every time the robotic wheelchair is over a landmark. To make this localization procedure functional, it is guaranteed that the robotic wheelchair attains a specific posture over the landmark. An entire metallic path connecting the initial and final points is not required but only segments of metallic paths. In order to guarantee a safe navigation, an obstacle avoidance strategy is also included. An adaptive dynamic trajectory-tracking controller is implemented to guarantee the asymptotic stability in the tracking control under heavy loads, which is the case of the combined user and wheelchair. Finally, experimental results obtained under many conditions are presented. The robotic wheelchair navigates without colliding

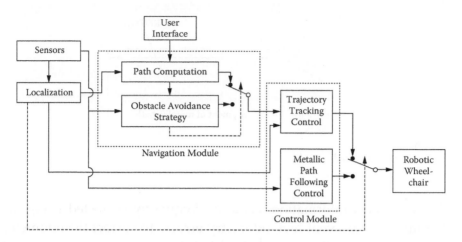

FIGURE 4.5
System architecture of the metallic tapes–based navigation.

through a very narrow doorway in one of the experiments. The experimental results show that the proposed navigation system is efficient and effective.

The proposed navigation system considers that the wheelchair navigates to the destination without any participation of the user in the control, as the navigation system is intended for people who have difficulties guiding a conventional wheelchair. The architecture of the wheelchair navigation system is illustrated in Figure 4.5. The user interface allows the user to choose on the PDA the destination using any of the following alternatives: eye blinks, eye-gaze movements, head or face movements, blowing and sucking, and brain waves, such as described in Chapter 3. The wheelchair localization is estimated using the information provided by inductive sensors, encoders, and an RFID reader. The path computation is generated using a topological map, a metric map, the current localization, and the destination requested by the user.

4.3.1 Localization of the Robotic Wheelchair

Odometry information (calculated using encoder signals) is used for localization of the wheelchair, which is corrected every time the wheelchair is over a landmark. Every landmark is composed of a segment of metallic path and an RFID tag. All landmarks are detected by inductive sensors and identified by an RFID reader (see Figure 4.3).

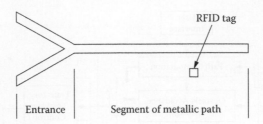

FIGURE 4.6
Segment of metallic path.

The odometry information has to be frequently corrected using the landmarks to prevent high odometry errors. To correct the odometry information, first, the robotic wheelchair is positioned over a segment of metallic path using a metallic path following controller and, second, when the wheelchair reaches the last of such segment of metallic paths, the odometry information is corrected, replacing it with the posture of the segment of metallic path. The posture of a segment of metallic path is defined by the position of the endpoint of the segment of metallic path and the orientation of such a segment of metallic path. Such procedures are described in detail in the next section.

4.3.2 Metallic-Path-Following Controller

The metallic-path-following controller is used to position the robotic wheelchair over a segment of metallic path, and a nonlinear control law is proposed for the metallic path following.

The basic segment of metallic path is shown in Figure 4.6. Every segment of metallic path has an entrance that is used to ensure that the inductive sensors detect a metallic path even if there are great errors on the trajectory tracking with respect to the real desired trajectory caused by odometry errors and control errors (see Figure 4.7).

To position the robotic wheelchair over a segment of metallic path means to position point h (Figure 4.7) at the middle line of this path.

A schematic of the robotic wheelchair and a metallic path are shown in Figure 4.8, where y_{wm} is the y_{wm}-axis component of coordinate <M>, which represents the position of point h with respect to the metallic path, and ψ_{wm} is the heading of the wheelchair relative to the x_{wm} axis of coordinate <M>. The metallic path is represented by a straight line (dashed line). Let us consider that the sign of y_{wt} can be measured, and

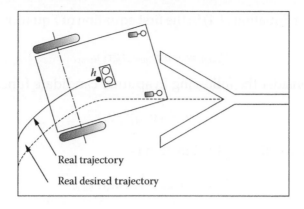

FIGURE 4.7
Robotic wheelchair going to the entrance of a metallic path segment. The real trajectory is the trajectory described by point *h* over the real workspace. The real desired trajectory is the trajectory that point *h* must follow over the real workspace.

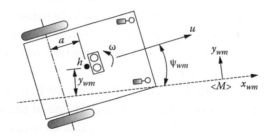

FIGURE 4.8
Schematic of the robotic wheelchair and a metallic path.

consider the following kinematic model of the wheelchair:

$$\dot{y}_{wm} = u \sin \psi_{wm} + a\omega \cos \psi_{wm}$$
$$\dot{\psi}_{wm} = \omega. \tag{4.2}$$

Assuming small values of ψ_{wm}, then Equation (4.2) can be approximated as follows:

$$\dot{y}_{wm} = a\omega$$
$$\dot{\psi}_{wm} = \omega. \tag{4.3}$$

The proposed nonlinear control law is

$$\omega = -K_{wm} \operatorname{sign} y_{wm} \tag{4.4}$$

where K_{wm} is a real variable greater than a positive value.

Replacing Equation (4.4) in the first equation of Equation (4.3) results in

$$\dot{y}_{wm} = -a\, K_{wm}\, \text{sign}\, y_{wm}. \tag{4.5}$$

Let us consider the following Lyapunov candidate function:

$$V = (y_{wm})^2 / 2.$$

The time derivative of this function is

$$\dot{V} = -y_{wm} a\, K_{wm}\, \text{sign}\, y_{wm},$$

which is negative definite by considering $a > 0$. Therefore, it is obtained that $y_{wm} \to 0$ as $t \to \infty$.

The sign of y_{wm} can be estimated by using the inductive sensors. If the left inductive sensor does not detect any metal and the right detects, then sign $y_{wm} = 1$. If the right inductive sensor does not detect any metal and the left detects, then $y_{wm} = -1$. If both inductive sensors detect metal, then sign $y_{wm} = 0$. If both inductive sensors do not detect any metal, the last sign of y_{wm} is used.

The variable K_{wm} uses two constants that switch according to the state of the inductive sensors is proposed. If one of the sensors detects a metal, then a small value of K_{wm} is used. If both sensors do not detect any metal, then a greater value of K_{wm} is used. The switch of K_{wm} improves the velocity of convergence because they converge faster when point h is more separated from the metallic path.

However, the control signal ω would switche in magnitude and sign, which may cause abrupt rotational accelerations. To obtain smoother rotational movements, the use of the following filter in the calculation of K_{wm} is proposed:

$$K_{wm} = \frac{\bar{K}_{wm}}{\lambda_{wm} S + 1}, \tag{4.6}$$

where $\bar{K}_{wm}$ is a switched constant as stated in the previous paragraph, and λ_{wm} is a constant greater than zero. The variable K_{wm} has to be set to a very small value greater than zero every time the sign of y_{wm} changes or passes through zero. Thus, small switching changes of ω are obtained under such situations. The stability conditions are preserved because K_{wm} remains greater than a constant greater than zero.

Let us consider the following property: If point h of the robotic wheelchair, which is at the front of the traction axis, follows a straight trajectory, the heading of the robotic wheelchair tends to the orientation of the straight trajectory. Therefore, if point h follows a straight metallic path, its heading will converge on the orientation of the metallic path.

A trajectory-tracking controller is used to drive the robotic wheelchair to the entrance of the segment of metallic path. Then, the metallic-path-following controller is turned on since at that instant both inductive sensors are on. Possibly, the inductive sensors could detect other segments of the metallic path that are over the desired trajectory, following a wrong metallic path. To prevent this error, the metallic-path-following controller is available only when the wheelchair is close to the target segment of the metallic path.

4.3.3 Correcting the Odometry Information

The RFID tag is placed on the floor (see Figure 4.6) such that the RFID reader on the rear of the wheelchair detects it when the inductive sensors are close to the final segment of metallic path. Since the instant that the RFID reader detects an RFID tag, the metallic-path-following controller is turned off and the robotic wheelchair continues its displacement, maintaining its last heading. The metallic-path-following controller is turned off to prevent the wheelchair from following the entrance to another segment of the metallic path (see landmarks 1 and 2 of Figure 4.9). When both inductive sensors are off, it is assumed that the inductive sensors have reached the final segment of metallic path. At this instant, the odometry information is updated with the posture information of the segment of metallic path identified by the RFID tag.

4.3.4 Topological Map

Every segment of metallic path and RFID tag defines a node of a directed graph. More specifically, the node is the posture of the segment of metallic path. The posture of a segment of metallic path is defined by the position of the endpoint of the segment of metallic path and the orientation of such a segment of metallic path. The graph defines a topological map. The segments of a metallic path are placed in several locations, specially in doorways, passageways, and target positions (see Figure 4.9). The current posture (initial point) and the final

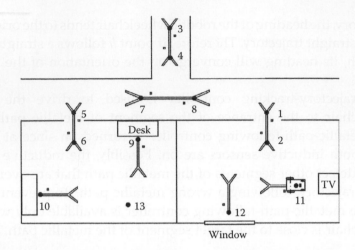

FIGURE 4.9
Distribution example of metallic path segments and RFID tags. Some segments of metallic path are superimposed as 1 and 2.

posture (final point) of the wheelchair do not need be over a segment of metallic path; nevertheless, these points are also considered to be nodes of the graph (see node 13 in Figure 4.9). The topological map is used to calculate a path from the initial point to the final point, ensuring that the wheelchair passes through a segment of metallic path in order to frequently correct the odometry.

The weights of the edges are calculated considering the estimated displacement that takes the robotic wheelchair between nodes—for example, the estimated displacement to go from node 10 to node 5 in Figure 4.9. To obtain better results, this estimated displacement could be calculated using path planning over a metric map. The displacement between two nodes is divided in two parts, where the first part corresponds to the displacement that takes the wheelchair from the initial landmark to the entrance of the goal landmark. The second part corresponds to the displacement of the wheelchair over the goal landmark. If the goal node has no landmark, the displacement only has the first part—that is, in this case, the displacement that takes the wheelchair from the initial node to the goal node. When the robotic wheelchair goes from one node to another node, it navigates using only the odometry information in the first part of the wheelchair displacement. To prevent high errors in the odometry, the following procedure is performed. When the estimation of the first part of the displacement

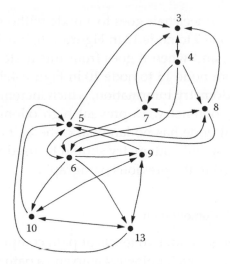

FIGURE 4.10
Example of the directed graph.

exceeds a limit, the corresponding edge is eliminated. Such a limit is called in this work the limit of the displacement using only odometry. In this case, an additional landmark may be required to connect the nodes whose edges were eliminated. Therefore, every time an edge is eliminated, the connectivity between the nodes of this edge has to be verified. For example, in Figure 4.10 the directed edge (10,8) is eliminated, but another landmark is not required because the nodes of this edge are connected through node 5. Another criterion to eliminate edges is the following. When navigation through unsafe passages is required between nodes, the corresponding edges should be eliminated. A narrow doorway is an example of unsafe passage, because the wheelchair may collide even though an obstacle avoidance strategy is used. For example, in Figure 4.10, the edge (7,5) is eliminated because to go from node 7 to node 5, first, the wheelchair has to reach the entrance of landmark 5, which implies the wheelchair has to go into the room through a narrow doorway. Based on these edge elimination criteria, the graph of Figure 4.10 is obtained from the schematic of Figure 4.9 considering only the left room.

The direct connection between two nodes without landmarks must be eliminated because, in this case, the wheelchair displacement using only odometry information can be unbounded, such as, when the robotic wheelchair navigates between these nodes indefinite times.

When the robotic wheelchair goes to a node without a landmark (for example, from node 9 to node 13 in Figure 4.9), it will use only odometry information, and when it goes from this node to any landmark (for example, from node 13 to node 10 in Figure 4.9), it will continue using only the odometry information, which increments the displacement using only odometry. To prevent high odometry errors when the initial or goal node has no landmark, the half of the limit of the displacement using only odometry should be used in the elimination criterion described in the previous paragraph.

4.3.5 Shortest Path Computation

In this navigation system, two levels of path computation are used: a path computation over a topological map and a path computation over a metric map. The first level corresponds to the search of the shortest path connecting multiple nodes of the topological map. The second level corresponds to the path planning between the position of a pair of nodes on such a topological map.

In the first level, the Dijkstra algorithm [14] on the graph corresponds to the topological map. In the second level, a shortest path over a metric map is generated. The initial position is the initial node position and the final position is a position close to the entrance of the goal segment of the metallic path. After the final position, a straight desired trajectory directed to the segment of metallic path is considered (see Figure 4.7). When the goal node has no landmark, a virtual landmark is generated with its virtual entrance. This is done only to obtain a straight trajectory before attaining the goal node. In the following subsection, the path planning between pairs of nodes corresponding to the second level of path computation is explained.

4.3.6 Path Planning Corresponding to the Second Level of the Path Computation

The following path-planning implementation is based on the basic path-planning structure [15] where a cell decomposition with fixed resolution is used to represent the environment, a graph using such a representation is generated, and over the graph the optimal path is obtained. Considering that the environment is a room or a passageway, which are small spaces, and/or considering a bounded separation

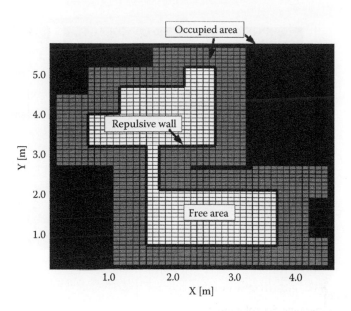

FIGURE 4.11
Preprocessed map.

between the positions of the nodes, a more sophisticated path-planning technique is not required.

The trajectory-planning system is separated in starting and trajectory-planning processes. The starting process takes into account a navigating environment discrete map where areas with and without obstacles are emphasized. Areas with obstacles are dilated according to the geometrical shape of the mobile vehicle. Figure 4.11 presents the result of such a preprocessing showing the separation of navigable and unnavigable cells with free and occupied areas, respectively. Finally, the occupied cells that form the repulsive wall are also separated. Thus, the following definition is created.

Definition 1: Let M be the set of all cells of a discrete metric map, which belong to at least one of the subsets C_F (free-cells set), C_B (occupied-cells set), and C_R (repulsive-cells set), so that $C_F \cup C_B = M$, $C_F \cap C_B = \emptyset$, and $C_B \cap C_R = C_R$.

So, the collision risk at each environment cell is defined as:

$$\begin{cases} c\,(cf) = \left(\dfrac{1}{K} \displaystyle\sum_{cr \in C_R} e^{-K_o \text{dist}(cf,cr)} \right) \times 100\% \\ c\,(cb) = 100\% \end{cases} \tag{4.7}$$

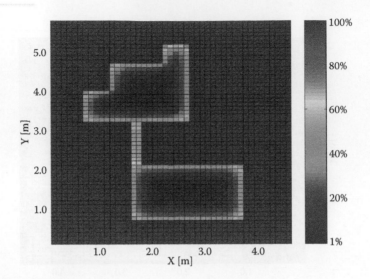

FIGURE 4.12
Collision-risk mapping. See color insert.

where $cf \in C_F$, $cb \in C_B$, $cr \in C_R$, K e is the number of repulsive cells, K_o is a positive constant, and $c\,(\cdot)$ is the collision risk established for each navigating environment cell. Figure 4.12 shows the collision-risk mapping obtained with Equation (4.7).

One can observe that while the process previously reported runs only once, the trajectory-planning process is executed so that a new initial or goal position is considered. The trajectory-planning process uses the initial and final positions of the mobile vehicle and the collision risk at each navigable cell of the environment. So, a path with the lowest collision risk connecting the initial position to the final position is generated by using the Dijkstra algorithm [14]. The Dijkstra algorithm calculates the shortest path in a graph. The graph used in this trajectory-planning process is generated as follows. Every node of the graph represents a free cell (see Figure 4.13). Every free cell is connected to its neighbor free cell and these connections are represented by edges in the graph. Finally, the weight of every edge is equal to the collision risk of the cell of whose node the edge points to. Such an algorithm also guarantees that the resulting path is the shortest among the most safe paths. Figure 4.14 presents the environment map with the generated path emphasized.

In the sequel, the centers of mass of the cells that form the path are interpolated through the spline-cubic interpolation method [16] and

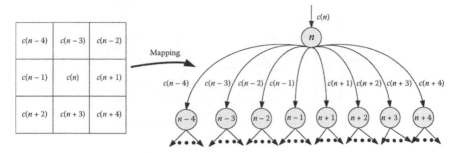

FIGURE 4.13
Graph generated from the discrete metric map.

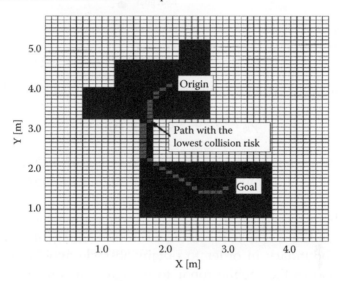

FIGURE 4.14
Environment map with generated path.

nonlinear sections are fitted by Bezier curves [17], resulting in a smooth and continuous path described by a polynomial.

4.3.7 Obstacle Avoidance

The obstacle avoidance strategy is based on the tangential escape approach [18], which was developed for position control of mobile robots. The tangential escape approach chooses an escape path that is tangent to the obstacle boundary. In order to obtain this tangent path, a virtual desired position is generated, rotating the real desired position with respect to the current mobile robot position.

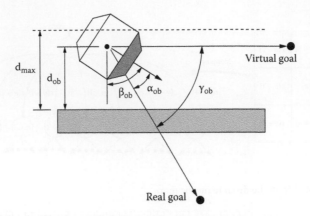

FIGURE 4.15
Mobile robot interacting with an obstacle.

The tangential escape strategy [18] is presented as follows:

$$\gamma_{ob} = \alpha_{ob} - \beta_{ob} + \operatorname{sign}(\beta_{ob})\frac{\pi}{2}, \tag{4.8}$$

where the angles α_{ob} and β_{ob} are shown in Figure 4.15 and d_{ob} is the distance of the robot to the obstacle. The angle γ_{ob} rotates the real goal to the new desired position (the virtual goal).

The characteristic of the tangential escape approach is that it is a simple solution to move the vehicle through a tangential path of the obstacle boundary in order to obtain obstacle avoidance. This approach allows the mobile robot to navigate in somewhat complex environments, as was stated in [18]. The considered complex environments in [18] are environments with many obstacles and environments where local minima are presented when using other methods such as impedance-based obstacle avoidance [19] [20]. The disadvantage of the tangential escape strategy proposed in [18] is that it was designed only for position control.

In the present section, a method that makes the tangential escape approach applicable to trajectory-tracking control is proposed. A laser scanner located at the front of the robotic wheelchair is considered. In the proposed method, a temporal desired position h_{dF} over the desired trajectory is defined when $d_{ob} <= d_{max}$ (see Figure 4.16), where d_{ob} is the least laser measurement and d_{max} is a constant. Thus, the tracking control over the original desired trajectory is turned off and a tracking control over a temporal desired trajectory is turned on. The temporal

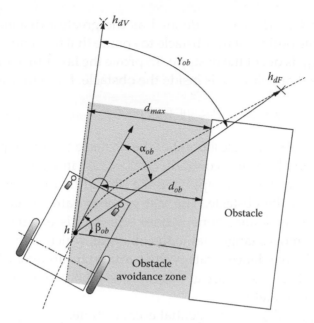

FIGURE 4.16
Robotic wheelchair interacting with an obstacle.

desired trajectory is a straight trajectory from the current wheelchair position to the temporal desired position h_{dF}. The temporal desired trajectory is used to obtain a constant velocity while the wheelchair goes to the temporal desired position. The procedure to obtain h_{dF} is described as follows:

1. Initiate $t_F = t_C$, where t_C is the last instant that the tracking control over the desired trajectory is active.

2. While $(\|h_d(t_F) - h(t)\| < (d_{max} + E_{pa})$ and $d_{ob} <= d_{max})$ make $t_F = t_F + T_s$. The variable E_{pa} is a positive constant and T_s is the sample time. All the loops of this step are performed in one sample time.

3. Repeat step 2 every sample time until the tracking control over the desired trajectory is turned on again.

In this procedure, t is the current time and h_d is the desired trajectory. Therefore, after applying step 2 of the last procedure, $h_{dF} = h_d(t_F)$. One can see from step 3 of the last procedure that h_{dF} could change every sample time.

The constant E_{pa} can be defined as the greatest distance between points of the outline of the obstacle to ensure that the temporal desired position h_{dF} is out of the obstacle. To prove the last affirmation, first let us assume that point h_{dF} is inside the obstacle. From this assumption,

$$\|h_{dF} - h\| \le \|h - P_{closest}\| + \|h_{dF} - P_{closest}\| < (d_{max} + E_{pa})$$

where $P_{closest}$ is the closest point of the obstacle outline to point h. The last inequality leads to a contradiction because inequality $\|h_{dF} - h\| \ge (d_{max} + E_{pa})$ results after applying the procedure to obtain h_{dF}. Then, h_{dF} is out of the obstacle. The last proof is valid when h is inside the obstacle avoidance zone, whose situation is obtained when the wheelchair moves tangential to the obstacle, which is the objective of the obstacle avoidance strategy. It is important to avoid having h_{dF} inside the obstacle because in this case the robot would go around the obstacle indefinitely.

When $d_{ob} \le d_{max}$, the tangential escape strategy is applied, rotating the temporal desired point h_{dF} in γ_{ob} degrees calculated from Equation (4.8), thus obtaining a virtual desired point h_{dV} (see Figure 4.16). When $d_{ob} > d_{max}$, the angle γ_{ob} is zero and point h_{dF} is maintained constant until point h is close to it. After h is close to h_{dF}, the trajectory tracking over the original desired trajectory is turned on again.

The tangential escape strategy is not applied ($\gamma_{ob} = 0$) when $|\beta_{ob} - \alpha_{ob}| > \pi/2$ because, in this case, the vehicle moves out of the obstacle avoidance zone when it goes to position h_{dF}.

In the robotic wheelchair, the laser sensor is at the front of the wheelchair and the control point h is at the middle of the wheelchair, which is different from common mobile robots where the control point and the laser sensor are at the middle of the robot. That causes differences in the behavior of the obstacle avoidance. In the second situation, the rotation of the robot does not cause a variation in the distance d_{ob}, but in the robotic wheelchair configuration, the rotation causes variation in the distance d_{ob}. When applying the obstacle avoidance strategy, the rotation of the wheelchair causes a positive variation of d_{ob}. That means that the front of the wheelchair is separating from the obstacle, which is good obstacle avoidance behavior.

One can observe that the angle γ_{ob} can vary abruptly when d_{ob} becomes less than d_{max} and vice versa. To solve this problem, γ_{ob} is smoothed using the following filter:

$$\dot{\bar{\gamma}}_{ob} = (\gamma_{ob} - \bar{\gamma}_{ob})/T_{ob}, \tag{4.9}$$

where T_{ob} is the rise time of the filter. The variable $\bar{\gamma}_{ob}$ is now used in the rotation of the goal position instead of γ_{ob}.

The movements of the robotic wheelchair in the obstacle avoidance strategy will be smoothed using the filter Equation (4.9). However, the velocity of the change of $\bar{\gamma}_{ob}$ may still be great. To improve the filter, the following system is used instead of Equation (4.9):

$$\dot{\bar{\gamma}}_{ob} = K_{ob} \tanh\left((\gamma_{ob} - \bar{\gamma}_{ob})/T_{ob}\right), \tag{4.10}$$

where K_{ob} is a constant greater than zero. Thus, K_{ob} will be the maximum value of $\dot{\bar{\gamma}}_{ob}$.

A laser scanner sensor is mounted in the front of the wheelchair, providing range measurements for the horizon of $180°$ ahead of it. Its position in the vehicle creates blind zones where it is not possible to detect obstacles, such as, for example, both sides of the wheelchair robot. Such blind zones may cause lateral collisions during vehicle rotation. To avoid such a collision, a circular trajectory with minimum radius is used (see Figure 4.17). The system shown in Equation (4.10) is used to obtain such a circular trajectory, since the minimum radius of the trajectory is equal to u/K_{ob}. The linear velocity u can be considered constant during the application of the obstacle avoidance strategy due to the definition of the temporal desired trajectory. However, the use of too small K_{ob} will cause problems when the obstacle is in front of the wheelchair. In this case, a greater K_{ob} is required to rotate faster in order to avoid the obstacle. Therefore, the following system can be used instead of Equation (4.10).

$$\dot{\bar{\gamma}}_{ob} = \begin{cases} K_{ob1} \tanh\left((\gamma_{ob} - \bar{\gamma}_{ob})/T_{ob}\right) & if \quad d|\bar{\gamma}_{ob}|/dt \geq 0 \\ K_{ob2} \tanh\left((\gamma_{ob} - \bar{\gamma}_{ob})/T_{ob}\right) & if \quad d|\bar{\gamma}_{ob}|/dt < 0 \end{cases}, \tag{4.11}$$

where K_{ob1} and K_{ob2} are constants greater than zero. The constant K_{ob1} is used when $|\bar{\gamma}_{ob}|$ is rising, which implies that a deviation of the wheelchair is required in order to avoid the obstacle. The constant K_{ob2} is used when $|\bar{\gamma}_{ob}|$ is decreasing, which implies that the wheelchair is tending to the temporal desired position h_{dF}. Therefore, $K_{ob1} > K_{ob2}$.

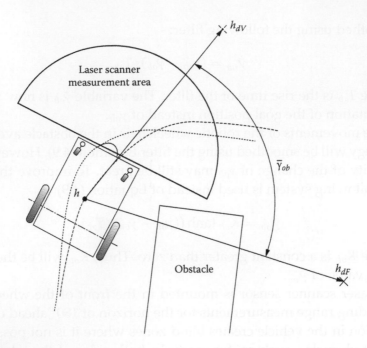

FIGURE 4.17
Obstacle inside the laser scanner's blind zone. The wheelchair will collide with the obstacle if it goes directly to the objective h_{dF}.

4.3.8 Switching Adaptive Control

In this section, the switching adaptive tracking and positioning control of a mobile robot, developed in [22], is described. This adaptive control is implemented in the navigation system presented here. The switching between parameter updating and nonparameter updating is used to avoid parameter drifting in the presence of measurement errors, noise, or disturbances. Constant model parameters as well as unknowns are considered.

4.3.8.1 Dynamic Model

A schematic of the robotic wheelchair is illustrated in Figure 4.18, where G is the center of mass; B is the wheel baseline center; $h = [x \ y]^T$ is the point that is required to track a trajectory; u and ω are the linear and angular velocities; ψ is the heading of the vehicle; and d, b, a are distances. One can see that the robotic wheelchair has the same structure as a unicycle-like mobile robot.

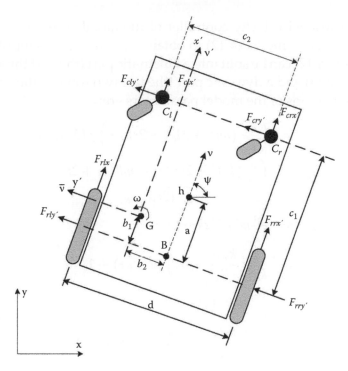

FIGURE 4.18
Schematic of the robotic wheelchair.

Let us consider the following dynamic model of a unicycle-like mobile robot [22] as the model of the robotic wheelchair:

$$
\begin{bmatrix} \dot{x} \\ \dot{y} \\ \dot{\psi} \\ \dot{u} \\ \dot{\omega} \end{bmatrix} = \begin{bmatrix} u\cos\psi - a\omega\sin\psi \\ u\sin\psi + a\omega\cos\psi \\ \omega \\ \dfrac{\theta_3^0}{\theta_1^0}\omega^2 - \dfrac{\theta_4^0}{\theta_1^0}u \\ -\dfrac{\theta_5^0}{\theta_2^0}u\omega - \dfrac{\theta_6^0}{\theta_2^0}\omega \end{bmatrix} + \begin{bmatrix} 0 & 0 \\ 0 & 0 \\ 0 & 0 \\ \dfrac{1}{\theta_1^0} & 0 \\ 0 & \dfrac{1}{\theta_2^0} \end{bmatrix} \begin{bmatrix} u_{ref} \\ \omega_{ref} \end{bmatrix} \qquad (4.12)
$$

where θ_i^0 is the ith model parameter and u_{ref} and ω_{ref} are the linear and angular reference velocities. Generally, these reference velocities are common input signals in commercial autonomous vehicles. Therefore, to maintain compatibility with other autonomous vehicles, it is useful to express the robotic wheelchair model in a suitable way by considering linear and angular reference velocities as control signals. The model of the low-level velocity controller of the mobile robot is considered inside dynamic model (4.12) to obtain u_{ref} and ω_{ref} as input signals. Equation (4.12) can be split into a kinematic part (the first three rows of the equation) and a dynamic part (the last two rows of the equation). The equations of the model parameters are:

$$\theta_1^0 = \left(\frac{R_a}{k_a} \left(mr^2 + 2I_e \right) + 2rk_{DT} \right) / (2rk_{PT}),$$

$$\theta_2^0 = \frac{\left(\frac{R_a}{k_a} \left(I_e d^2 + 2r^2 \left(I_z + mb^2 \right) \right) + 2rdk_{DR} \right)}{(2rdk_{PR})},$$

$$\theta_3^0 = \frac{R_a}{k_a} mbr / (2k_{PT}), \tag{4.13}$$

$$\theta_4^0 = \frac{R_a}{k_a} \left(\frac{k_a k_b}{R_a} + B_e \right) / (rk_{PT}) + 1,$$

$$\theta_5^0 = \frac{R_a}{k_a} mbr / (dk_{PR}),$$

$$\theta_6^0 = \frac{R_a}{k_a} \left(\frac{k_a k_b}{R_a} + B_e \right) d / (2rk_{PR}) + 1$$

where m is the system mass (wheelchair and its user); I_z is the wheelchair's moment of inertia around the vertical axis located at G; r is the right and left wheel radius; k_b is the voltage constant of the electric motors multiplied by the gear ratio; R_a is the electric resistance constant of the electric motors; k_a is the torque constant of the electric motors multiplied by the gear ratio; I_e and B_e are the moment of inertia and the viscous friction coefficient of the combined motor rotor, gearbox, and wheel; k_{PT} and k_{DT} are the proportional and derivative (PD) gains of the linear velocity PD control of the robotic wheelchair; and k_{PR} and k_{DR} are the proportional and derivative gains of the angular velocity PD control of the robotic wheelchair. As one can see in (4.13), the model parameters θ_i^0 are functions of mass and moment of inertia of the wheelchair with user, motor parameters, and low-level PD control parameters.

The linear parametrization of the dynamic part of (4.12) is [22]:

$$\begin{bmatrix} \dot{u} & 0 & -\omega^2 & u & 0 & 0 \\ 0 & \dot{\omega} & 0 & 0 & u\omega & \omega \end{bmatrix} \theta^0 = \begin{bmatrix} u_{ref} \\ \omega_{ref} \end{bmatrix}, \tag{4.14}$$

where $\theta^0 = [\theta_1^0 \quad \theta_2^0 \quad \ldots \quad \theta_6^0]^T$. Rearranging, it results that

$$D\dot{v} + T_a \theta^0 = v_{ref} \tag{4.15}$$

where

$$D = \begin{bmatrix} \theta_1^0 & 0 \\ 0 & \theta_2^0 \end{bmatrix}, \quad v = \begin{bmatrix} u \\ \omega \end{bmatrix}, \quad v_{ref} = \begin{bmatrix} u_{ref} \\ \omega_{ref} \end{bmatrix},$$

$$T_a = \begin{bmatrix} 0 & 0 & -\omega^2 & u & 0 & 0 \\ 0 & 0 & 0 & 0 & u\omega & \omega \end{bmatrix}. \tag{4.16}$$

4.3.8.2 Adaptive Control

Let us consider the following tracking and positioning adaptive control [21]:

$$v_{ref} = \hat{D}M(v - N) + T_a\hat{\theta} \tag{4.17}$$

$$v = \ddot{h}_d + K_1\dot{\tilde{h}} + K_2\tilde{h}, \qquad \tilde{h} = h_d - h \tag{4.18}$$

$$\dot{\hat{\theta}} = K_A Y^T P e_T, \tag{4.19}$$

where

$$M = \begin{bmatrix} \cos\psi & \sin\psi \\ -\frac{1}{a}\sin\psi & \frac{1}{a}\cos\psi \end{bmatrix},$$

$$N = \begin{bmatrix} -u\omega\sin\psi - a\omega^2\cos\psi \\ u\omega\cos\psi - a\omega^2\sin\psi \end{bmatrix}, \tag{4.20}$$

$\hat{\theta}$ is an estimate of the true parameters vector θ^0, $\hat{D}$ is matrix D defined with estimated parameters instead of true parameters, h_d and $\dot{h}_d$ define the desired trajectory, $K_1 \in \mathbb{R}^{2\times 2}$ and $K_2 \in \mathbb{R}^{2\times 2}$ are diagonal positive definite matrices,

$$h = \begin{bmatrix} x \\ y \end{bmatrix}, \tag{4.21}$$

$$e_T = \begin{bmatrix} \tilde{h} \\ \dot{\tilde{h}} \end{bmatrix}, \quad Y = \begin{bmatrix} 0 \\ \hat{M}^{-1}T \end{bmatrix} \in \mathbb{R}^{4\times 6} \tag{4.22}$$

$$T = \begin{bmatrix} T_{11} & 0 & -\omega^2 & u & 0 & 0 \\ 0 & T_{22} & 0 & 0 & u\omega & \omega \end{bmatrix}, \tag{4.23}$$

$$\begin{bmatrix} T_{11} \\ T_{22} \end{bmatrix} = M(\ddot{h} - N), \tag{4.24}$$

$$\hat{M} = \hat{D}M. \tag{4.25}$$

The parameter a (see Figure 4.18) must be non-null to avoid singularities in the control signals. The acceleration $\ddot{h}$ of Equation (4.24) has to be estimated based on the measured velocities. The constant matrix $K_A \in \mathbb{R}^{6 \times 6}$ is a diagonal matrix defined such that $K_A > 0$ and matrix $P \in \mathbb{R}^{4 \times 4}$ is defined as follows: $P = P^T > 0$ such that

$$A_K^T P + P A_K = -Q; \quad Q = Q^T > 0 \tag{4.26}$$

where

$$A_K = \begin{bmatrix} 0 & I \\ -K_2 & -K_1 \end{bmatrix}, \tag{4.27}$$

and I is a 2×2 identity matrix.

Matrix A_K is Hurwitz because K_1 and K_2 are diagonal matrices with positive elements different from zero. Therefore, if matrix P is calculated from Equation (4.26), using some $Q = Q^T > 0$, then one can obtain a matrix P such that $P = P^T > 0$.

From Equation (4.22) it can be observed that to compute Y one has to avoid $\hat{\theta}_1 = 0$ and $\hat{\theta}_2 = 0$. To do this, a projection algorithm is applied:

$$\hat{\theta}_i = l_i \quad if \quad \hat{\theta}_i \le l_i - \zeta_i \tag{4.28}$$

where $i = 1, 2$; l_i is the minimum possible value of θ_i^0; $\zeta_i > 0$; and $l_i - \zeta_i > 0$. This projection algorithm is defined considering $\theta_i^0 > 0$ for $i = 1, 2$. The objective of this algorithm is to maintain $\hat{\theta}_i$ with $i = 1, 2$ between acceptable values. The values l_i with $i = 1, 2$ can be chosen knowing the identified parameter values of similar systems.

4.3.8.3 Switching Strategy

The switching strategy switches between adaptive and nonadaptive laws, in order to avoid parameters drifting in the presence of measurement errors, noise, or disturbances.

The adaptive law works as an integrator and, therefore, it can cause robustness problems in case of measurement errors, noise, or disturbances. One possible way to prevent parameter drifting is by turning off the parameter updating when the control error is smaller than a boundary value, as shown in [23]. The same idea is used in [21] but with a switching control approach.

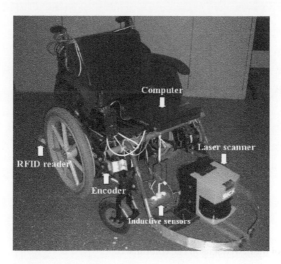

FIGURE 4.19
Robotic wheelchair of UFES/Brazil.

The proposed switching strategy is as follows:

$$\dot{\theta}^{+}(t) = \begin{cases} \dot{\theta}(t) & \text{if} \quad V_{eT}(t) > C_v \\ 0 & \text{if} \quad V_{eT}(t) \le C_v \end{cases} \qquad (4.29)$$

where

$$V_{eT} = e_T{}^T P e_T, \qquad (4.30)$$

and C_v is a constant greater than zero.

4.3.9 Hardware

The hardware architecture of the robotic wheelchair (Figure 4.19) consists of: (1) a commercial powered wheelchair from which only the mechanical structure and motors are used; the power card and joystick are discarded; (2) two encoders directly connected to the motors; (3) an MSP430F1611 microcontroller from Texas Instruments where the low-level velocity control is implemented; (4) a power card that amplifies pulse-width modulation (PWM) signals obtained from the microcontroller and sends them to the motors; (5) a computer where the high-level control algorithms are implemented; (6) inductive sensors; (7) an RFID reader; and (8) a laser scanner. The high-level control algorithms are implemented under a Windows operating system using Microsoft Visual C++.

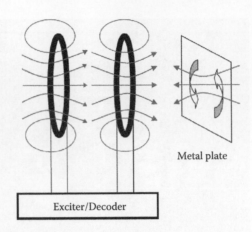

Metal plate

Exciter/Decoder

FIGURE 4.20
Schematic view of inductive sensor. See color insert.

The inductive sensors detect, through electric fields, the proximity to metallic objects, such as aluminium, copper, and others. Each inductive sensor is composed of two LC circuits that are made of two similar coils axially aligned and fastened around an air core (see Figure 4.20). The coils are separated by a distance equal to their radius, guaranteeing a weak magnetic coupling between them. The differential detection and reading with multiple sample techniques are implemented to deal with the external magnetic fields, electromagnetic waves, and electric fluctuations in the circuit.

In the differential detection, the metal plate is detected by a decoder comparing the relative voltages on the LC circuits, providing a great immunity to many kinds of fluctuations in the circuit caused by voltage supply variations, electric noise, and others. Figure 4.20 presents the magnetic fields of two coils with the same polarity. In this configuration, over the influence of an electromagnetic noise of a distant source, one can consider that the field of the electromagnetic noise goes through both coils with similar intensity. That will result in similar induction in both coils with practically null difference in the inducted voltage and the consequent elimination of the noise by the differential factor of the detection process. It is important to consider that the electromagnetic noises closer to the sensor are inside the physical dimensions of the robotic wheelchair. Thus, this noise source can be relocated. For example, there are in the robotic wheelchair high electromagnetic noise sources such as power cables that supply switching current to the motors. The following was verified experimentally. When these power cables are 5 cm from the sensor, the sensor is unable to operate. However, when the power cables are 20 cm from the sensor (current configuration of the robotic wheelchair), the electromagnetic noise caused by this source is practically eliminated.

The reading with multiple samples techniques consider that several sources of electric and magnetic noise are of a transitory nature. The detection cycle of the sensor is designed to treat these transient noises by a process of multiple samples and discards. The detection cycle performs four excitations, in which the three last samples are considered to validate the readings. The reading is valid when the three last samples are equal. Thus, high immunity to noise is obtained, without great detriment to the sensibility. More than 1,000 complete detection cycles per second were performed and there was no considerable delay in the detections.

4.3.10 Experiments

Several experiments were carried out with the robotic wheelchair described in the previous section.

The parameters used in the navigation system are presented in the following. The parameters of the switching adaptive control are:

$$K_1 = \begin{bmatrix} 6 & 0 \\ 0 & 6 \end{bmatrix}, \quad K_2 = \begin{bmatrix} 0.5 & 0 \\ 0 & 0.5 \end{bmatrix},$$

$$K_A = diag(1/32, 1/32, 1/80, 1/5, 1/0.8, 1/0.16),$$

$$l_{l1} = 0.14, \quad l_{u1} = \infty, \quad l_{l2} = 0.7, \quad l_{u2} = \infty, \quad (4.31)$$

$$l_{l3} = -\infty, \quad l_{u3} = \infty, \quad l_{l4} = 0.9, \quad l_{u4} = 1.2,$$

$$l_{l5} = -0.03, \quad l_{u5} = 0.03, \quad l_{l6} = 0.9, \quad l_{u6} = 1.2,$$

$$C_v = 0.005,$$

where $diag(.)$ represents a diagonal matrix.

The parameter a of the kinematic part of the robotic wheelchair model in Equation (4.12) is chosen as 0.35 m. The initial estimated model parameters used in the switching adaptive control are as follows:

$$\hat{\theta}_1^0 = 0.3308, \quad \hat{\theta}_2^0 = 0.1317, \quad \hat{\theta}_3^0 = -0.0152,$$

$$\hat{\theta}_4^0 = 1.0144, \quad \hat{\theta}_5^0 = 0.0712, \quad \hat{\theta}_6^0 = 0.8944. \quad (4.32)$$

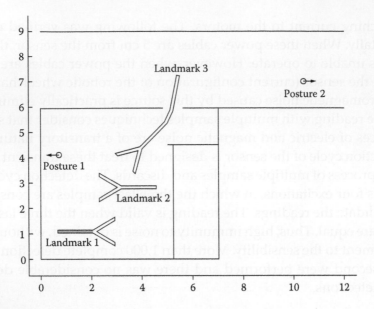

FIGURE 4.21
Schematic of the environment considered in the experiments.

These identified model parameters correspond to a robotic wheelchair without a user. The identification of the robotic wheelchair model was performed by using least squares estimation [24] applied to a filtered regression model [25] obtained from Equation (4.14).

From Equation (4.6), the parameters of the metallic-path-following controller are:

$$K_{wm} = \begin{cases} 0.2 & \text{if one of the inductive sensors is on} \\ 0.6 & \text{if both of the inductive sensors are off/on} \end{cases}$$

$$\lambda_{wm} = 0.5.$$

The parameters of the obstacle avoidance strategy are:

$$d_{max} = 1.2, \quad E_{pa} = 2, \quad T_{ob} = 3$$

$$K_{ob1} = 1.5, \quad K_{ob2} = 0.4.$$

Figure 4.21 shows the schematic of the environment considered in the experiments, which is a representation of a metric map and the locations of the landmarks and two objectives.

Figure 4.22 illustrates the directed graph that represents the topological map of the environment shown in Figure 4.21.

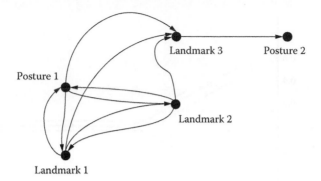

FIGURE 4.22
Directed graph of the environment considered in the experiments.

The result of the metallic-path-following control is illustrated in Figure 4.23. The final position of the segment of metallic path is reached by the wheelchair; specifically, control point h (see Figure 4.8) reaches the end of the segment of metallic path. In addition, the heading of the wheelchair reaches the orientation of the segment of metallic path. The described trajectory of the wheelchair is smooth and convergent to the metallic path. This smooth convergence can also be observed

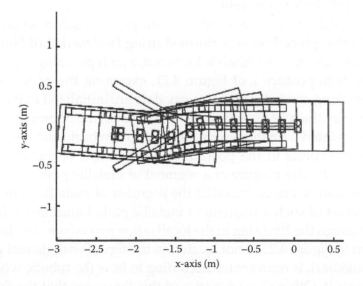

FIGURE 4.23
Evolution of the metallic-path-following control. The wheelchair goes from left to right. The red line is the trajectory described by control point h.

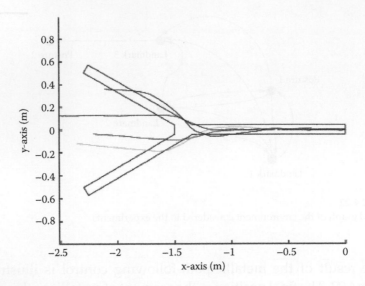

FIGURE 4.24
Trajectories described by four cases of the metallic path following control by the wheelchair with users of 78 kg, 100 kg, 62 kg, and 78 kg of weight, respectively.

in Figure 4.24, which shows the results of four cases of metallic-path-following control that were executed with different users of 62 kg, 78 kg, and 100 kg of weight.

Figure 4.25 shows the results of a simple navigation where, first, a localization procedure is performed using landmark 2 of Figure 4.21. After the robotic wheelchair is localized, a path planning is performed and goes to posture 1 of Figure 4.21, executing the adaptive trajectory tracking control. The odometry data are initialized in the posture (0,0,0) after the robotic wheelchair is localized, the odometry information is updated with the posture (4.54,2.84,0) (wheelchair in Figure 4.25 that corresponds to the posture of the segment of metallic path of landmark 2). The posture of a segment of metallic path is defined by the position of the endpoint of the segment of metallic path and the orientation of such a segment of metallic path. Landmark 2 is identified through the RFID tag in the localization procedure. The landmark shown in Figure 4.25 is not located in the figure with its real posture; this landmark is represented according to how the robotic wheelchair perceives it. Other characteristics of this figure are that the described trajectory by the wheelchair is reconstructed using the odometry information, and the corrected odometry posture is represented by the

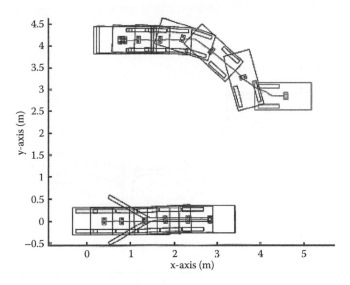

FIGURE 4.25
Robotic wheelchair navigation: localization with landmark 2 and reaching the posture 1.

wheelchair. These three characteristics of Figure 4.25 are also observed in the following figures corresponding to other experiments.

Figure 4.26 shows the results of a navigation where the robotic wheelchair returns to landmark 2 from posture 1. The initial wheelchair posture and the initial odometry information are the last wheelchair posture and the last odometry information of the previous experiment. After the wheelchair reaches the end of landmark 2, the odometry is corrected with the posture (4.54,2.84,0) (green wheelchair in Figure 4.26).

An experiment of a navigation from the same landmark used in the previous experiments to another objective (posture 2 of Figure 4.21) was performed. The results of this experiment are shown in Figure 4.27. An intermediate landmark must be used to go through a narrow doorway. The short-path computation determines this path based on the topological map of Figure 4.22. One can see that a direct connection from landmark 2 to posture 2 is not allowed because an unsafe passage is presented in this path and also the displacement using only odometry is too large, which may cause great odometry errors.

In the following experiments, three cases of robotic wheelchair navigation are performed. All of these experiments are navigation from landmark 1 to posture 2 of the environment shown in Figure 4.21. The

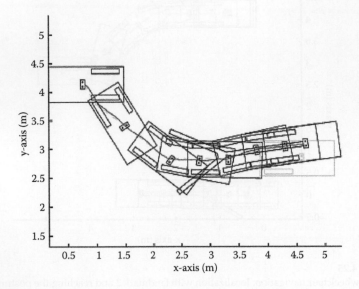

FIGURE 4.26
Robotic wheelchair navigation: reaching landmark 2 from posture 1.

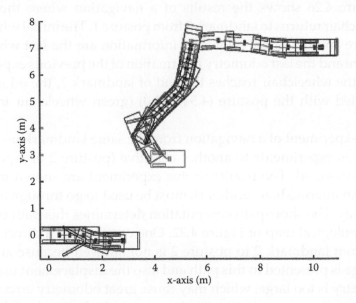

FIGURE 4.27
Robotic wheelchair navigation: localization with landmark 2 and reaching the posture 2.

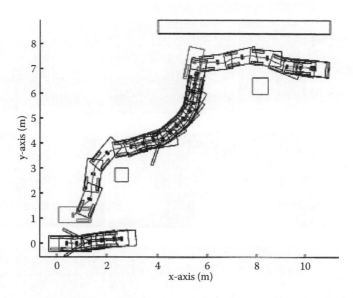

FIGURE 4.28
First case of the robotic wheelchair navigation performed from landmark 1 to posture 2.

results of these experiments are shown in Figures 4.28 to 4.33. Figures 4.29 to 4.31 show a sequence of photos corresponding to the first of these experiments. Different positions of the obstacles are used in these experiments. The first of these experiments is performed with a user of 78 kg and the rest are performed with a user of 62 kg. One can observe that in all of these experiments a successful navigation is performed avoiding obstacles, going through a narrow doorway, and reaching the objective. The robotic wheelchair goes through the narrow doorway, using the metallic-path-following controller, with a velocity of 0.075 m/s.

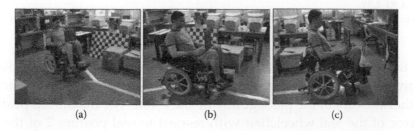

(a)　　　　　　　　　(b)　　　　　　　　　(c)

FIGURE 4.29
Robotic wheelchair navigation. Part 1: Localization with landmark 1. See color insert.

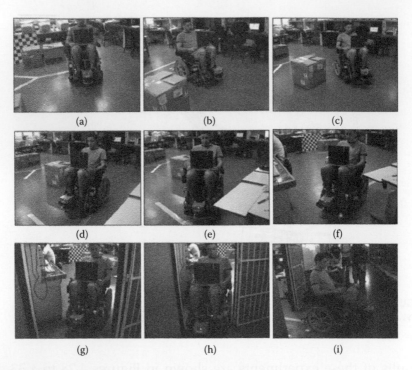

FIGURE 4.30
Robotic wheelchair navigation. Part 2: reaching landmark 3 avoiding an obstacle. See color insert.

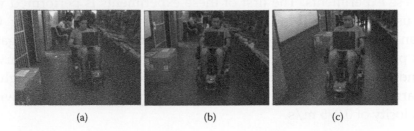

FIGURE 4.31
Robotic wheelchair navigation. Part 3: reaching posture 2 avoiding an obstacle. See color insert.

Based on the experimental results, one can see that the final posture can be specified to be over the end of a segment of metallic path or any other posture in the passageway or the room. The maximum position error of the real wheelchair with respect to real posture 2 of the last four experiments is 45 cm and the mean of these errors is 17.75 cm; all these position errors were measured using a tape measure. As one

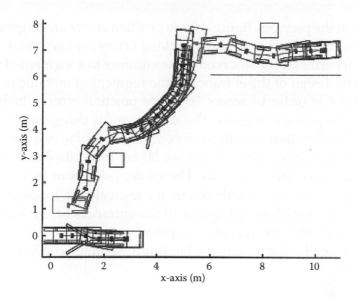

FIGURE 4.32
Second case of the robotic wheelchair navigation performed from landmark 1 to posture 2.

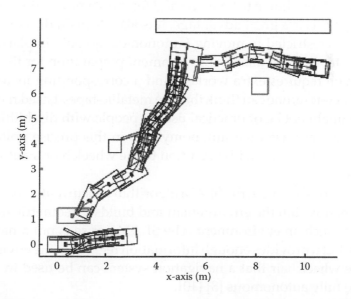

FIGURE 4.33
Third case of the robotic wheelchair navigation performed from landmark 1 to posture 2.

can see in the previous figures, these position errors are largely caused by odometry errors because the tracking errors are very small. Similar odometry errors were observed at the entrance to a segment of metallic path. The design of the entrance of the segment of metallic paths was performed in order to accept 50 cm of position error, which can be seen in the previous figures. The displacement using only odometry is less than 6 m. Based on these experimental results, one can consider that the odometry error is less than 50 cm for a displacement using only odometry less than 6 m. Therefore, using 6 m as the limit of the displacement using only odometry to create the topological map, the robotic wheelchair will attain all the entrances of the segments of metallic path that are over the computed path. This conclusion allows a robust localization because a landmark is attained every time it is required.

4.4 SLAM-Based Navigation

As shown in the previous section, metallic-tapes-based navigation systems have been shown to be successful for indoor navigation purposes. Although this is a great advantage, it is also its main drawback, since the user is restricted to moving (autonomously) only in places where metallic tapes are available. Environment preparation for this type of navigation requires extra workers and a corresponding increment of costs. Therefore, one can think that the metallic-tapes-based navigation system might not be of practical use for people with disabilities, since it does not increase their autonomy. It is in this precise point where the SLAM can offer a wider solution to the wheelchair's autonomous navigation.

As previously stated, the SLAM algorithm concurrently localizes the wheelchair within the environment and builds a geometric model—a map—of such an environment. The SLAM per se is not a navigation system, but it provides enough information regarding the environment and the wheelchair that a navigation system can be used in order to become fully autonomous [8] [10].

The SLAM algorithm implemented is an EKF (Extended Kalman Filter) based approach that extracts corners and walls from the environments (associated with point-based and line-based features [12] [1]).

The feature extraction procedure is achieved by using laser range data acquired by the laser sensor implemented in the footrest of the wheelchair, as shown in Figure 4.3.

We have used the SLAM algorithm for two main objectives: to acquire precise information of unknown surrounding environments, and to use such information for risky maneuvers. However, it is worth mentioning that before using a SLAM algorithm, its consistency must be properly checked [10], due to the fact that the error associated with the SLAM estimation process will be propagated to all the stages that use the SLAM (e.g., the control strategy and the planning stage). The behavior of the error associated with the estimation process is valuable information that will allow us to know how precise the maneuver that the user intends to perform needs to be, or if the available information is enough for actually performing a risky maneuver, always taking into account that the user must be protected.

The SLAM algorithm uses the range readings—from the laser sensor mounted on the footrest of the wheelchair, as shown in Figure 4.3—to concurrently localize the wheelchair within the environment and to build a geometric model—a map—of such an environment. The latter is achieved by the implementation of an EKF (Extended Kalman Filter) based SLAM that extracts corners—concave and convex—and lines—associated with walls—from the environment. The programming and optimization issues, and consistency results of the implemented EKF-SLAM, can be found in a previous work of the authors [26][27]. It is worth mentioning that the SLAM algorithm is an approach that can be used by a navigation strategy to enhance its performance.

4.4.1 Obtaining an Accurate Map

Considering that the aim of the SLAM algorithm is to build a map of the surrounding environment, such an algorithm performs as a secondary process where a user modality interface drives the wheelchair's motion, as shown in Figure 4.34. An implemented example of this situation can be found in [26].

In Figure 4.34, the user commands the wheelchair's motion through one of the modalities previously presented. The control commands as well as the laser sensor readings from the environment are the inputs of the EKF-SLAM algorithm [27]. The SLAM algorithm returns the

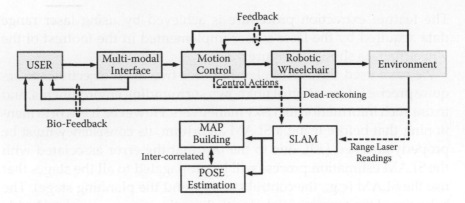

FIGURE 4.34
Scheme of the SLAM algorithm as a secondary process during navigation.

instantaneous position of the wheelchair within the environment and a map of such an environment.

Thus, the SLAM algorithm is used only to model the environment that surrounds the wheelchair's navigation and to estimate the wheelchair's position. It is worth mentioning that the map of the environment and the position of the wheelchair within that environment are obtained from the SLAM system state [27]. Furthermore, the SLAM algorithm is activated once the user selects the semiautonomous navigation option shown in Figure 4.34.

Figure 4.34 shows how the SLAM algorithm is implemented on the navigation system. As can be seen, the SLAM algorithm behaves as a secondary—but parallel—process of the navigation system. It acquires the laser range readings, the dead reckoning from the wheelchair, and the motion control commands to perform a consistent and concurrent estimation of the wheelchair's position and the environment, in real time [8]. One of the main advantages of the SLAM algorithm is that once the wheelchair has navigated an environment, the obtained map can be stored on the onboard computer and used later for navigational purposes. The map obtained receives a tag name under which it is stored. If the user revisits the same environment, then the map can be uploaded and the user will be able to select any navigable point within the map, as shown in [13]. A path-following controller will then guide the motion of the wheelchair.

Figure 4.35 shows an example of a map obtained from the EKF-SLAM algorithm. The points are raw laser data, and the solid segments

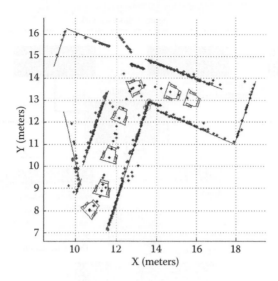

FIGURE 4.35
Example of map obtained by the EKF-SLAM implemented.

are associated with extracted lines from the environment, whereas the circles are the detected corners. The dotted line is the path traveled by the robotic wheelchair [27].

4.4.2 Managing Risky Maneuvers

Based on the SLAM system state, information regarding the environment surrounding the robotic wheelchair is available. Such information is used for two specific cases: crossing a door and turning within passageways. Both situations, although trivial, require great effort of the wheelchair's user. The crossing-a-door problem requires precision, whereas the turning process requires both precision and information regarding backward movements. The SLAM algorithm, in this case, provides the necessary information to perform both processes properly.

The crossing-a-door problem is summarized in Figure 4.36 [1]. This system architecture can be briefly summarized as follows:

- The human–machine interface (shown in the previous chapter) receives the user's signals and generates motion commands to the robotic wheelchair. In addition, the interface communicates to the user when a door has been detected. If more than one door

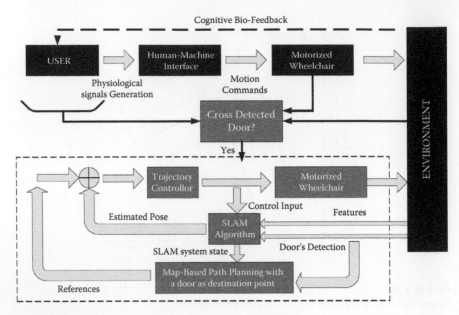

FIGURE 4.36
General architecture of the SLAM-based crossing-a-door solution.

is detected, the interface allows the user to choose which door to cross. The latter is accomplished by means of the same signals used to command the wheelchair's motion [27]. If no door is chosen to cross, then the wheelchair motion control remains under the user's decision. It is worth mentioning that the user's control stage is closed by a cognitive biofeedback loop based on both the environment information and the perception of the wheelchair motion according to the user [27].

- The laser range sensor mounted on the wheelchair's footrest, shown in Figure 4.3, is used to acquire the information regarding the surrounding environment. The raw range data acquired by the sensor is processed for door detection and environmental features extraction. Specifically, the door-detection procedure is based on the histogram method [26], which obtains the Cartesian position of the door with respect to a reference frame attached to the vehicle. The features extracted from the environment correspond to lines (associated with walls) and corners (convex and concave). The detected doors and the features acquired from the environment are used by the SLAM algorithm. It is worth mentioning that the positions of the detected doors are also part of the SLAM system state and are used for localization purposes of the wheelchair.

- The map estimated by the SLAM algorithm is used for planning purposes. The Frontier Points Method [1] is used to locally plan a feasible and safe path between the wheelchair's position and the middle point of the door chosen by the user. The Frontier Points Method guarantees that a collision-free path can be found within the mapped environment. Such a path is updated at each sampling time of the SLAM algorithm. The reference path generated by the path-planning stage is compared to the vehicle's estimated position, and such a comparison is fed to the trajectory controller. The trajectory controller used is an adaptive trajectory controller with exponential stability [1].

If the user chooses to cross the detected door, then the control of the wheelchair switches to the trajectory controller. Hence, the crossing-a-door problem is performed autonomously. The SLAM algorithm starts once the user chooses a detected door from the environment. After crossing the detected door, the SLAM memory usage is released from the onboard computer. In addition, the onboard system allows for the detection of multiple doors, and the user decides which door to cross. Figure 4.37 shows a visualization of the interface and the three possible door morphologies that the system is able to detect.

In addition, Figure 4.38 shows two experimental results of the cross-a-door system developed [1]. As can be seen, the system detects the doors, plans a feasible path from the wheelchair's position up to the middle point of the door, and the path-tracking control system drives the vehicle until reaching the door's middle point.

Finally, the SLAM algorithm used in this approach is an EKF-based SLAM, which extracts corners and walls (associated with lines) from the environment, in order to construct a Cartesian map of the surrounding environment [1].

The second SLAM-based risky maneuver is a turning strategy that allows the user of the wheelchair to autonomously reach a desired orientation within a narrowed environment. This approach is useful for people who have muscle spasms or loss of muscle activity, due to the great effort they have to make in order to perform backward movements. Briefly, the turning strategy uses the SLAM-based map for planning a suitable and safe collision-free path to be followed, autonomously, by the robotic wheelchair. Details of this implementation can be found in [27] [10]. The method can be summarized as follows:

1. A visual interface allows the user to choose the desired orientation.

2. The computational system uses the map built by the SLAM algorithm and the estimate of the wheelchair position within

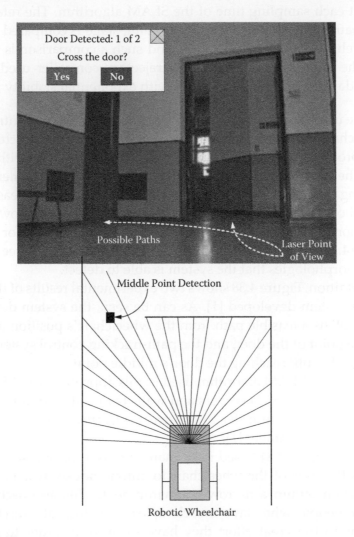

FIGURE 4.37
Door-detection interface and three cases of environment morphology for doors' detection. See color insert for (a). *(Continued)*

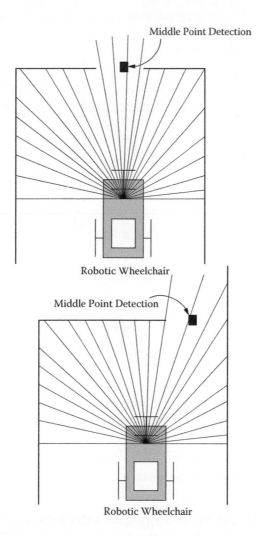

FIGURE 4.37

(Continued). Door-detection interface and three cases of environment morphology for doors' detection. See color insert for (a).

the environment to check if there is enough space available for a safe navigation.

3. Following, a Monte Carlo–based semicircle generation searches for the minimum cost path based on the successive generation of semicircles of variable radius, as shown in Figure 4.39 [27].

4. Once a path is found, a trajectory controller drives the wheelchair until it reaches a neighborhood of the desired orientation.

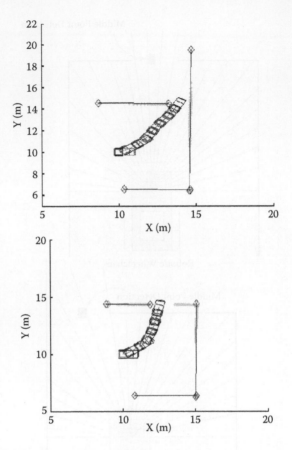

FIGURE 4.38
Experimental results of the cross-a-door problem.

The proposed turning strategy guarantees the existence of a solution. Further details of this method can be found in [27]. Additionally, Figure 4.39 shows an example of the turning strategy. In this figure, the desired orientation is 180 degrees from the current wheelchair's orientation, useful for passageway navigation; the initial orientation of the wheelchair is $\theta = 1.4$ rads. The solid dark square represents the wheelchair within the environment; the solid green lines represent the successively feasible paths found by the system, whereas the solid magenta path is the one chosen as the optimum (according to a cost criterion presented in [27]). The solid gray segments are associated with lines extracted from the environment, whereas the solid blue rectangle circumscribes the map in order to restrict the maneuverability area. As can be seen, all feasible paths ensure a safe turning.

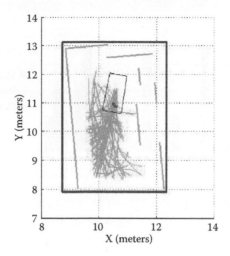

FIGURE 4.39
Example of the turning strategy. See color insert.

Once a path is chosen, the same trajectory controller presented in [26] is implemented to drive the wheelchair's motion until reaching the desired orientation.

4.5 Statistical Results

Despite the fact that the autoguided mode of the robotic wheelchair is intended to improve the user's capabilities, such a mode needs to be evaluated by a greater population. The experimental tests shown here were conducted by a seven-person population with different disabilities [4]. Briefly, all volunteers agreed that the modality had improved their mobility; however, the volunteers expressed their lack of comfort in using the autonomous navigation approach, mainly due to their possible lack of confidence in unmanned vehicles. Two points from the questionnaire filled out by the patients are worth mentioning in this section [4]:

- Do you think that this modality has improved your mobility? [Score between 3 (for high improvement) and 0 (unacceptable improvement)].

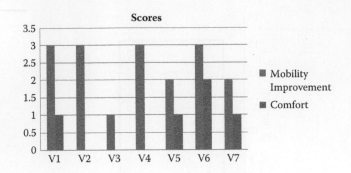

FIGURE 4.40
Example of the turning strategy.

- Did you feel comfortable using this modality? [Score between 3 and 0 (for not comfortable at all)].

Figure 4.40 shows the statistical results for these two questions. As can be seen, most patients do not feel comfortable with the autonomous system, although they recognize that it has improved their mobility, as stated in [4].

4.6 Semiautonomous Navigation

As a closure to this chapter, we would like to emphasize that the results shown in Figure 4.40 open a door for a new kind of human–machine interface. In Chapter 3, we presented a user-dependent interface for commanding the robotic wheelchair. On the other hand, in Chapter 4, we have presented an autoguidance system for driving the robotic wheelchair. However, the user does not feel comfortable with this approach and such results must be taken into account. Therefore, we believe—and from the best of our knowledge—that hybrid architectures are the answer: The user should be able to command the robotic wheelchair by his/her own means, but the wheelchair should also be able to perform tasks autonomously. Moreover, crossing a door or turning back maneuvers should be performed autonomously although the user must retain a certain level of control on such processes.

References

[1] F Auat Cheein, C De la Cruz, T Bastos, R Carelli, *SLAM-based cross-a-door solution approach for a robotic wheelchair*, Int. J Adv Robot Syst, Vol. 6, 2009.

[2] F Martins, W Celeste, R Carelli, M Sarcinelli, T Bastos, *An adaptive dynamic controller for autonomous mobile robot trajectory tracking*, Control Eng Pract, Vol. 16, 2008.

[3] F Auat Cheein, C De la Cruz, R Carelli, T Bastos, *Silla de ruedas robotizada con navegación autónoma asistida para entornos restringidos*, Revista Iberoamericana de Automática e Informática Industrial, Vol. 8 (2), 2011.

[4] T Bastos, F Auat Cheein, S Muller, W Celeste, C De la Cruz, D Cavalieri, M Saricinelli, P Amaral, E Perez, C Soria, R Carelli, *Towards a new modality-independent interface for a robotic wheelchair*, IEEE Trans Neural Syst Rehabil Eng, Vol. 90, p. 1–16, 2013.

[5] F Auat Cheein, N Lopez, F di Sciasio, F Lobo Pereira, R Carelli, *SLAM algorithm applied to robotic assistance for navigation in unknown environments*, J Neuroeng Rehabil, Vol. 7 (10), 2010.

[6] Y Hagiwara, T Shoji, H Imamura, *Position and rotation estimation for mobile robots in outside of recording path using ego-motion*, IEEJ T Electron, Inform Syst, Vol. 133 (2), 2013.

[7] B Wang, Z Li, W Ye, Q Xie, *Development of human-machine interface for teleoperation of a mobile manipulator*, Int. J Control Autom Syst, Vol. 10 (6), 2012.

[8] F Auat Cheein, *SLAM-based maneuverability strategy for unmanned car-like vehicles*, Robotica, Vol. 31, 2013.

[9] J Guivant, E Nebot, *Optimization of the simultaneous localization and map-building algorithm for real-time implementation*, IEEE T Robot Autom, Vol. 17 (3), 2001.

[10] F Auat Cheein, R Carelli, *Unmanned Robotic Service Units in Agricultural Tasks*, IEEE Indust Electron, forthcoming, 2013.

[11] F Auat Cheein, F Lobo, F di Sciascio, R Carelli, *Autonomous local-ization and mapping driven by Monte Carlo uncertainty maps-based navigation*, Knowl Eng Rev, Vol. 28 (1), 2013.

[12] F Auat Cheein, G Steiner, G Perez, R Carelli, *Optimized EIF-SLAM algorithm for precision agriculture mapping based on visual stems de-tection*, Comput Electron Agr, Vol. 78, 2011.

[13] F Auat Cheein, R Carelli, W Celeste, T Bastos, F di Sciascio, *Maps managing interface design for a mobile robot navigation governed by a BCI*, J Phys: Conference Series, Vol. 1 (10), 2007.

[14] A S Tanenbaum, *Computer Networks*, vol. 1, 4th ed., Prentice Hall, USA, 2003.

[15] S S Ge, F L Lewis, *Autonomous Mobile Robots: Sensing, Con-trol, Decision Making and Applications*. CRC Taylor and Francis, 2006.

[16] G D Knott, *Interpolating Cubic Splines: Progress in Computer Science and Applied Logic*. Birkhuser, Boston, 1999.

[17] L Shao, H Zhou, *Curve fitting with bezier cubics*. Graph Model Im Proc, Vol. 58, pp. 223–232, 1996.

[18] A Ferreira, W C Celeste, F A Cheein, T F Bastos-Filho, M Sarcinelli, R Carelli, *Human-machine interfaces based on EMG and EEG applied to robotic systems*, J Neuroeng Rehabil, Vol. 5 (10), 2008.

[19] N Hogan, *Impedance control: An approach to manipulation*, J Dyn Syst, T ASME, Vol. 107, pp. 1–23, 1985.

[20] H Secchi, R Carelli, V Mut, *Discrete stable control of mobile robots with obstacles avoidance*, International Conference on Advanced Robotics, pp. 405–411, 2001.

[21] C L Cruz, R Carelli, T F Bastos-Filho, *Switching adaptive control of mobile robots*, International Symposium on Industrial Electronics, pp. 835–840, 2008.

[22] C L Cruz, R Carelli, *Dynamic model based formation control and ob-stacle avoidance of multi-robot systems*, Robotica, Vol. 26 (3), pp. 346–356, 2008.

[23] F N Martins, W C Celeste, R Carelli, M Sarcinelli-Filho, T F Bastos-Filho, *Kinematic and adaptive dynamic trajectory tracking controller for mobile robots*, International Conference on Advances in Vehicle Control and Safety, pp. 29–34, 2007.

[24] K J Aström, B Wittenmark, *Adaptive Control*, 2nd ed. Addison-Wesley, pp. 199–223, 1995.

[25] F Reyes, R Kelly, *On Parameter Identification of Robot Manipulator*, International Conference on Robotics and Automation, pp. 1910–1915, 1997.

[26] F A Cheein, R Carelli, W C Celeste, T F Bastos-Filho, F D Sciascio, *Maps managing interface design for a mobile robot navigation*, J Phys: Conference Series, Vol. 90, p. 012088, 2007.

[27] F A Cheein, C L Cruz, T F Bastos-Filho, R Carelli, *Slam-based cross-a-door solution approach for a robotic wheelchair*, Int J Adv Robot Syst, Vol. 6 (3), pp. 239–248, 2009.

[28] F Wolfe, *A brief clinical health assessment instrument: Clinhaq*, Arthritis Rheum, Vol. 32, p. C49, 1989.

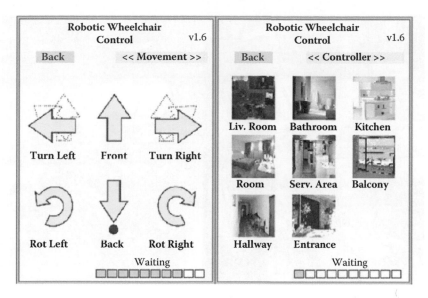

COLOR FIGURE 3.2
Different options of movement commands (arrows of movement or symbols representing places) presented on the PDA screen onboard the wheelchair.

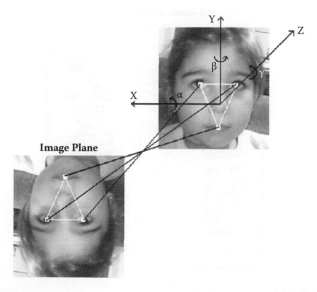

COLOR FIGURE 3.5
Facial features.

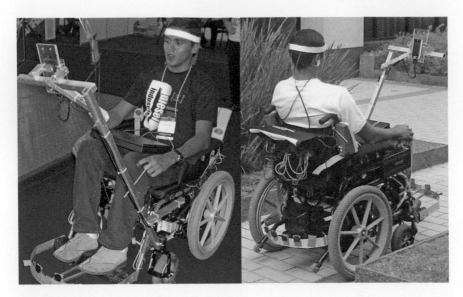

COLOR FIGURE 3.11
Robotic wheelchair commanded by mental tasks.

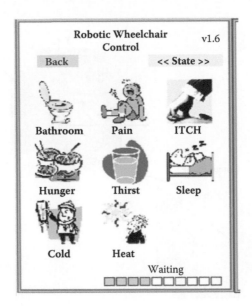

COLOR FIGURE 3.14
Options for communication: (a) letter to make sentences; (b) icons representing feelings or wishes.

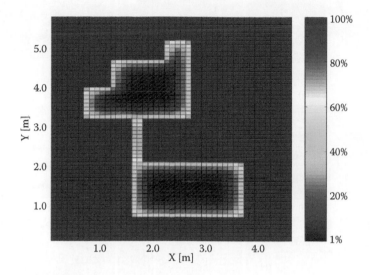

COLOR FIGURE 4.12
Collision-risk mapping.

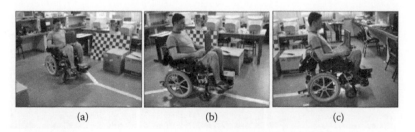

(a)   (b)   (c)

COLOR FIGURE 4.29
Robotic wheelchair navigation. Part 1: Localization with landmark 1.

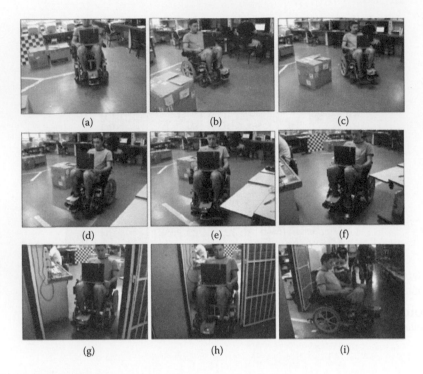

COLOR FIGURE 4.30
Robotic wheelchair navigation. Part 2: reaching landmark 3 avoiding an obstacle.

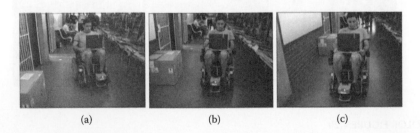

COLOR FIGURE 4.31
Robotic wheelchair navigation. Part 3: reaching posture 2 avoiding an obstacle.

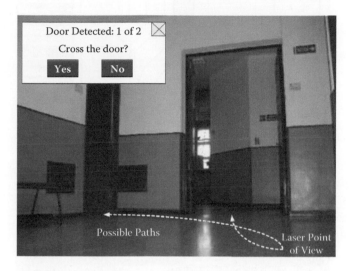

Door Detected: 1 of 2

Cross the door?

Yes   No

Possible Paths

Laser Point of View

COLOR FIGURE 4.37
Door-detection interface and three cases of environment morphology for doors' detection.

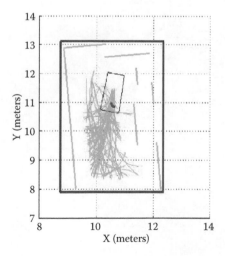

COLOR FIGURE 4.39
Example of the turning strategy.

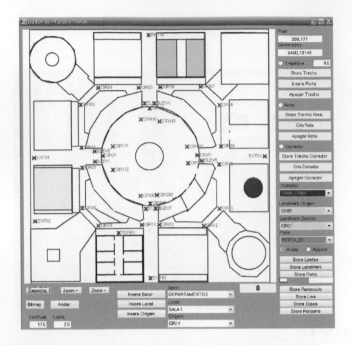

COLOR FIGURE 5.14
Screenshot of the accessibility information XML files editor.

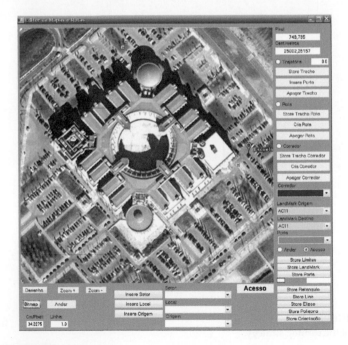

COLOR FIGURE 5.15
Edition of the building geographic position information screen.

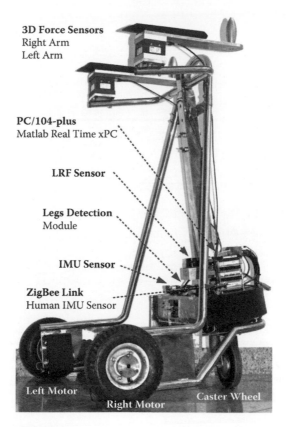

COLOR FIGURE 6.2
Details of UFES Smart Walker.

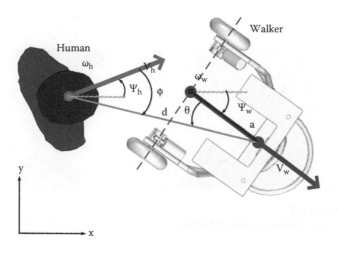

COLOR FIGURE 6.3
Kinematic model used for the controller of UFES Smart Walker.

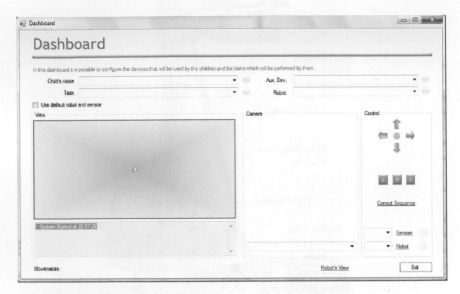

COLOR FIGURE 7.1
Main screen of the system.

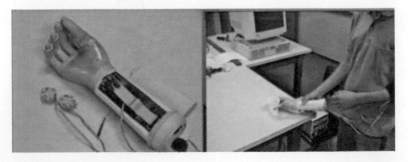

COLOR FIGURE 8.5
Myoelectric prosthesis developed in UFES/Brazil, which has force and temperature sensors.

5

Assisted Route Planner for a Robotic Wheelchair

Mariana Rampinelli Fernandes, Paulo Amaral, Raquel Frizera Vassallo, and Teodiano Freire Bastos-Filho
Universidade Federal do Espírito Santo, Brazil

Daniel Pizarro, Juan Carlos Garcia, and Manuel Mazo
Universidad de Alcala, Spain

CONTENTS

5.1 Introduction

For people with disabilities, some everyday tasks and situations can present physical constraints very hard to be overcome by them. In this case, wheelchairs are standard devices that can help them increase their locomotion ability and life quality. However, it is very difficult for a wheelchair user to plan the necessary movements in a place never visited before. These difficulties are mainly due to the lack of accessibility information [1] ensuring that there is a possible way for a wheelchair to go from the entrance to a desired location in a building. For outdoor navigation, a common solution [2] [3] [4] is the use of high-precision systems and databases like GPS (Global Positioning System) and GIS (Geographic Information System). The intention is to provide a navigation system to wheelchair users that could display, in real time, accessibility information that allows a safe motion between locations in open environments.

For indoor navigation, GPS positioning information is usually hard to obtain. The largest research and development effort aims to give autonomous behavior to a wheelchair in order to move from one location to another. Several works in the literature try to apply mobile robotics techniques using 3D sensors (video cameras and laser range finders) for determining the wheelchair location and automatic mapping of the environment using SLAM (Simultaneous Localization and Mapping) techniques, such as shown in the previous chapter.

Another area of research proposes the creation of smart spaces, removing from the wheelchair and placing in the environment the capacity of processing/sensing needed to generate the information and plans for navigation in the environment [5] [6]. In [7] a navigation system is proposed where the environment is modeled based on a hierarchically structured tree using the architectural features of the building. In that work, the navigation relies on information provided by optical encoders coupled to the wheelchair's motors. The wheelchair position calibration is based on video cameras and visual landmarks placed in doors and halls. On the other hand, [8] proposes an autonomous navigation system in small areas for a wheelchair using technologies applied to AGV (Automatic Guided Vehicles) and maps fetched from a local server. The location system of the wheelchair is based on an external radio system, and the route-planning algorithm is left to the local server.

In [6] a navigation method for service mobile robots in indoor environments is introduced. That method uses semantic maps encoded in XML (eXtensible Markup Language) and sensors placed in the smart space for the wheelchair location. Those maps describe the features of the multiple cells, their points of connection, and the location sensors in each one, simplifying the routing tasks.

This chapter presents the use of cameras and beacons in a smart space for the wheelchair location, and a simple and efficient tool that allows the retrieval of the accessibility information in public or private buildings, shopping centers, airports, companies, and so forth to help the autonomous navigation of a robotic wheelchair in those kinds of indoor environments. The accessibility information of a particular building is provided by an Internet service. Administrators of buildings and public places can store in the Internet server the accessibility information in the form of XML files that contain the description of floors maps, access points, places of interest, and optimal routes for a wheelchair to move inside the building. Wheelchair positions and identification of sites the wheelchair is passing by can be corrected using visual marks placed on the ceiling. A complete structure is proposed allowing autonomous navigation of a wheelchair in buildings, from any point outside on a sidewalk to any place of interest, on any floor of the building, and also between locations within the same building. It also presents an editor for XML files containing metric maps and accessibility information, and shows a control program for a wheelchair to fetch these files from the server using a cell phone. With the maps and accessibility information retrieved from the XML files, it controls the wheelchair for autonomous navigation within the building.

5.2 Wheelchair Indoor Navigation System Architecture

Figure 5.1 shows the main components and functions of the wheelchair indoor navigation system architecture here proposed. At the top left corner an Internet server is shown, which is dedicated to the storage of the XML files containing the maps and accessibility information. Creation, maintenance, and updating of this information can be done offline, even in a different location (shown in the top right corner of Figure 5.1). At the bottom, the embedded control system onboard the wheelchair is shown. The system behaves as follows: When approaching a certain location of interest, the wheelchair control system sends to the Internet server its geographical position (obtained from a GPS) through a mobile phone and then it gets information from registered buildings nearby. Then, the user selects the desired building and gets its XML files with the maps and the accessibility information to be used by the navigation system.

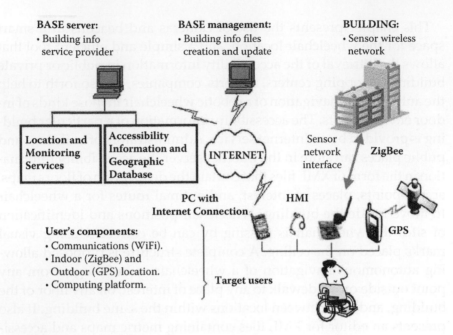

FIGURE 5.1
Architecture of the indoor wheelchair navigation system.

The choice of locations to be visited may be done by any of the different modalities previously presented. The selection is made using the appropriate modality, depending on the user's capabilities. Communication and positioning structures of the navigation system can be used for remote monitoring of biological signals and location of wheelchair users, opening a broad range of possible health care services.

5.2.1 Localization of the Robotic Wheelchair in a Smart Space

The intelligent space built at UFES/Brazil has two labs of 60 m² each and a corridor that links them. Eleven cameras are installed in the intelligent space; the corridor has three cameras and each lab has four cameras. All cameras are model DBK21AUC03, manufactured by the Imaging Source, and each one has a CMOS color sensor with resolution equal to 750 × 480 pixels, frame rate up to 75 fps, and is connected to each serve through a USB cable. The robotic wheelchair used in this work is manufactured by Freedom. Figure 5.2 shows the structure of the intelligent space.

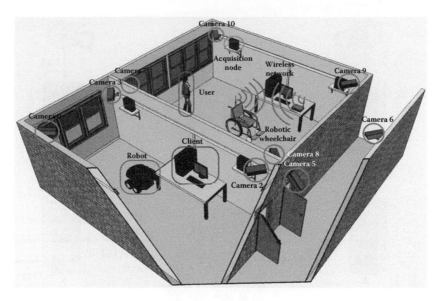

FIGURE 5.2
3D structure of the intelligent space.

5.3 Distributed Architecture for Acquisition and Processing

Implementing intelligent spaces requires a system capable of acquiring and processing data provided by a set of cameras fixed in the laboratories and in the corridor. It is important to mention that the image grabbing must be synchronized. Thus, a client–server architecture that allows the capture and processing of the images has been implemented.

Each camera is controlled by a processing node, the server, which acquires the images through the acquisition bus, in this case the USB. Low-level image processing is performed in this node, such as the identification on the image of the wheelchair marks. In each one of these acquisition and processing nodes, a TCP/IP server that gives the obtained information from each image to the client has been implemented.

Such a client, the one that implements the final part of the algorithm, is responsible for gathering the data provided by the servers, recovering the 3D wheelchair position and sending the movement commands to the wheelchair, which also implements a TCP/IP server through the wireless link. The whole system has been developed in high-level

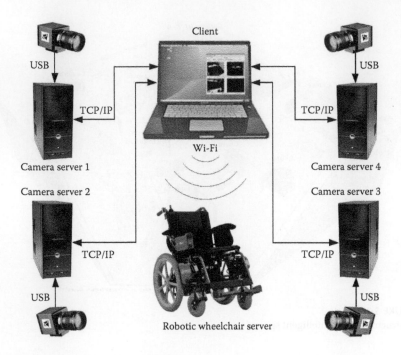

FIGURE 5.3
Architecture of the intelligent space's communication.

programming language C++. The communication architecture of the intelligent space is presented in Figure 5.3.

The identification of the robotic wheelchair in the intelligent space is done by three beacons built with infrared LEDs positioned on the top of the robot, forming a right triangle. Even in critical illumination conditions, those beacons make the wheelchair localization easier and also simplify the image-processing algorithm. The estimate of the vehicle's position is performed by finding the beacons' center of mass in the images. The infrared LEDs were chosen due to an important feature of this kind of application: the emission pattern, which must be as bright as possible to facilitate its localization, no matter the angle between the cameras and the wheelchair.

Since the cameras used in the intelligent space do not have an infrared filter, the detection algorithm becomes simpler by taking into consideration two important features: an infrared LED will appear as a circle in the image and as a high-saturation white color blob. The implementation is based on [9] and due to its simplicity, the computational

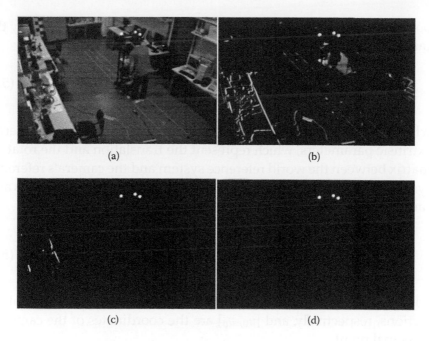

FIGURE 5.4

Steps to robotic wheelchair localization in the intelligent space: (a) original image; (b) background subtraction result; (c) thresholded image; and (d) classified objects in image.

cost is low. The general steps of the implemented algorithm are:

- background subtraction
- image segmentation
- identifying the beacons and extracting important features (area, perimeter, and eccentricity)
- classifying the selected points

These steps are illustrated in Figure 5.4. From three detected points that represent the mobile robot, it is possible to determine its coordinates and orientation in the 3D space.

5.4 Camera Model and 3D Reconstruction

The pinhole camera model defines the geometric relationship between a 3D world point P and its 2D projection onto image plane. This relationship can be described by Equation (5.1), which relates the 3D world point $\mathbf{P} = [X, Y, Z]^T$ to its pixel position $\mathbf{p}_i = [u_i, v_i, 1]^T$ viewed by the camera i.

$$\lambda \begin{bmatrix} u_i \\ v_i \\ 1 \end{bmatrix} = \mathbf{K}_i \begin{bmatrix} \mathbf{R}_i \begin{bmatrix} X \\ Y \\ Z \end{bmatrix} + \mathbf{T}_i \end{bmatrix}, \tag{5.1}$$

where the vector $\mathbf{T}_i = [T_{x_i}, T_{y_i}, T_{z_i}]^T$ and the matrix $\mathbf{R}_i$ are the camera's extrinsic parameters, which represent the translation and the rotation matrix between the world reference system and the camera's reference system. The matrix $\mathbf{K}_i$ contains the camera's intrinsic parameters and can be written as

$$\mathbf{K}_i = \begin{bmatrix} f_{x_i} & 0 & u_{0_i} \\ 0 & f_{y_i} & v_{0_i} \\ 0 & 0 & 1 \end{bmatrix}, \tag{5.2}$$

where f_u and f_v are the focal distance on horizontal and vertical directions, respectively, and $[u_0, v_0]$ are the coordinates of the camera's principal point.

After the camera servers detect the beacons of infrared LEDs in each captured image by each camera in the intelligent space, the 3D reconstruction of the robotic wheelchair can be achieved on the client. This way, the reconstruction is implemented with the triangulation algorithm described in [9] [10], which uses two or more images of the same scene, but captured by different cameras at the same time. It is noteworthy that the intrinsic and extrinsic cameras' parameters, described in Section 5.4, must be known in order to use this algorithm.

Considering the 3D point $\mathbf{P}$ viewed by two calibrated cameras i and j like $\mathbf{p}_i$ and $\mathbf{p}_j$, as shown in Figure 5.5. By using the Equation (5.1), it is possible write $\mathbf{P}$ using the two cameras' parameters as

$$\begin{bmatrix} X \\ Y \\ Z \end{bmatrix} = \lambda_i \mathbf{R}_i^{-1} \begin{bmatrix} \frac{u_i - u_{0_i}}{f_{x_i}} \\ \frac{v_i - v_{0_i}}{f_{y_i}} \\ 1 \end{bmatrix} - \mathbf{R}_i^{-1} \mathbf{T}_i = \lambda_i \mathbf{R}_i^{-1} \mathbf{r}_i - \mathbf{R}_i^{-1} \mathbf{T}_i, \tag{5.3}$$

and

$$\begin{bmatrix} X \\ Y \\ Z \end{bmatrix} = \lambda_j \mathbf{R}_j^{-1} \begin{bmatrix} \frac{u_j - u_{0_i}}{f_{x_j}} \\ \frac{v_j - v_{0_i}}{f_{y_j}} \\ 1 \end{bmatrix} - \mathbf{R}_j^{-1} \mathbf{T}_j = \lambda_j \mathbf{R}_j^{-1} \mathbf{r}_j - \mathbf{R}_j^{-1} \mathbf{T}_j, \tag{5.4}$$

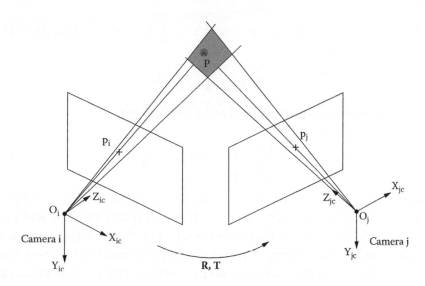

FIGURE 5.5
Point P in 3D world frame viewed by two calibrated cameras, *i* and *j*.

where the indices i and j designate the parameters of cameras i and j, respectively. Once point **P** is the same to both cameras, it is possible to combine Equations (5.3) and (5.4) as

$$\lambda_i \mathbf{r}_i = \lambda_j \mathbf{R}_{ij} \mathbf{r}_j - \mathbf{T}_{ij}, \tag{5.5}$$

where

$$\mathbf{R}_{ij} = \mathbf{R}_i \mathbf{R}_j^{-1}$$
$$\mathbf{T}_{ij} = \mathbf{R}_i \mathbf{R}_j^{-1} \mathbf{T}_j + \mathbf{T}_i.$$

The matrices $\mathbf{R}_{ij}$ and $\mathbf{T}_{ij}$ are composed of a series of transformations. First, the point **P** viewed in the image plane j is converted into a point on the world reference system. Then, this same point is converted from the world reference system into the image plane i. In this way, these transformations implement a direct transformation between the image plane j and i. Thus, Equation (5.5) can be written in matrix form as

$$\begin{bmatrix} -\mathbf{R}_{ij}\mathbf{r}_j, & \mathbf{r}_i \end{bmatrix} \begin{bmatrix} \lambda_j \\ \lambda_i \end{bmatrix} = \mathbf{T}_{ij}. \tag{5.6}$$

Writing $\mathbf{A} = [\ -\mathbf{R}_{ij}\mathbf{r}_j, \quad \mathbf{r}_i \ ]$ and $\mathbf{x} = [\ \lambda_j, \quad \lambda_i \ ]^T$, Equation (5.6) can be written as

$$\mathbf{Ax} - \mathbf{T} = 0. \tag{5.7}$$

The solution to Equation (5.7) can be found by

$$\mathbf{x} = \begin{bmatrix} \lambda_j \\ \lambda_i \end{bmatrix} = (\mathbf{A}^T\mathbf{A})^{-1}\mathbf{A}^T\mathbf{T}, \tag{5.8}$$

where only λ_i and λ_j are unknown values. Thereby, the 3D world point **P** can be obtained by using these values in Equations (5.3) and (5.4). Whether the influence of the errors is excluded, the coordinates of point **P** calculated by Equations (5.3) and (5.4) would match. However, there are errors in calibration and image processing. Then, those values are generated within a zone of uncertainty. To solve this problem, it is assumed that the errors involved in the process are identical for both cameras. Thus, the average point generated by the arithmetic mean of the results of each camera is taken as a reference.

5.5 Experiments

This section presents a comparison between the robot's positions obtained from the tracking system developed and those supplied by the odometry system of the robot. The experiments were performed in a laboratory with four fixed cameras and four TCP/IP camera servers connected by an Ethernet link. The experiments are separated in two categories: straight and curved paths. In the first case, the robot was commanded to follow a straight path. For each 900 mm, an image was acquired from each camera. Seven images were taken from each camera for each path. In the second experiment, the robot performed a curved path that resembles a step.

5.5.1 Experiment 1—Straight Path

In this stage, the robot was commanded to perform a straight path, as shown in Figure 5.6, repeating it five times. Figure 5.7 shows manual, odometry, and computer vision measures of the robot's position to one

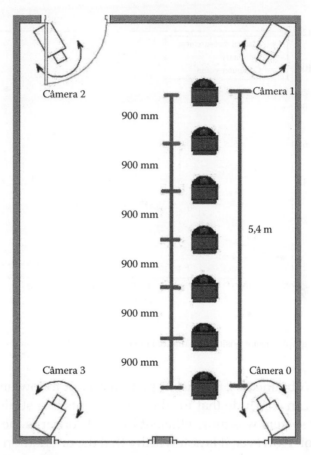

FIGURE 5.6
Straight path performed by the robot.

of these experiments, and Tables 5.1 and 5.2 describe the statistics data generated from the comparison between the obtained values.

In all experiments, the measures obtained by using computer vision were more similar to those obtained by manual measurement, as shown in Figure 5.7, which also can be observed in Table 5.1. In this table, it is possible to notice that the MSE (mean square error) value obtained with computer vision is 4.5 times smaller than the one obtained with odometry. The same happens to the standard deviation.

Regarding orientation data collected in Table 5.2, the values of the MSE and standard deviation are smaller for the odometry system. Analyzing the correlation, the values obtained with odometry follow the pattern of the values obtained with manual measurement while

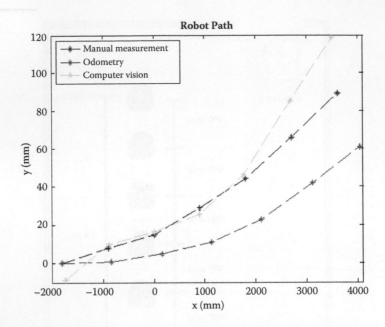

FIGURE 5.7
Experiment 1 graph—robot position by manual measurement, odometry, and computer vision.

the values obtained by the vision system do not follow any behavior. Then, we can conclude that for the experiments in a straight line, the odometry system was more efficient in what concerns the orientation of the robot. However, it is noteworthy that the orientation of the robot in this experiment is zero, or very close to it, since the path is straight. Therefore, even though there is a slight variation of the orientation obtained by the vision system as observed by MSE and standard deviation of Table 5.2, the correlation obtained a negative value. Moreover, the good performance of odometry could be due to the good accuracy achieved by the robot's gyroscope.

5.5.2 Experiment 2—Curved Path

In this experiment, the robot was commanded to follow a curved path, as shown in Figure 5.8, repeating it five times. Figure 5.9 shows manual, odometry, and computer vision measurements of the robot's position to one of these experiments, and Tables 5.3 and 5.4 describe the statistics data generated from the comparison between the obtained values.

In all experiments, the robot's position obtained by using computer vision were more similar to those obtained by manual measurement, as

TABLE 5.1

Analysis of Robot Position: Comparison Between Odometry and Computer Vision Measurement by Mean Square Error (MSE), Standard Deviation, and Correlation With the Manual Measurement.

		Odometry (mm)	Vision (mm)
Path 1	MSE	197.9	43.31
	Standard Deviation	158.5	29.94
	Correlation	0.9986	1.000
Path 2	MSE	204.4	48.78
	Standard Deviation	161.4	36.61
	Correlation	0.9980	0.9999
Path 3	MSE	195.5	41.33
	Standard Deviation	158.2	34.42
	Correlation	0.9985	0.9999
Path 4	MSE	213.9	43.64
	Standard Deviation	167.9	25.97
	Correlation	0.9988	1.000
Path 5	MSE	200.7	41.25
	Standard Deviation	154.7	31.01
	Correlation	0.9988	1.000

shown in Figure 5.7, which also can be observed in Table 5.3. It is possible to notice that the MSE value obtained with computer vision is 4.3 times smaller than the one obtained by odometry, for all experiments. The same can be noticed for standard deviation.

Regarding the orientation data, shown in Table 5.4, the values obtained of the MSE and standard deviation are very close to vision and odometry systems in all experiments.

5.6 Maps and Accessibility Information Modeling in XML Files

Building maps and accessibility information should include the existing locations to be visited, the best entry point, the best path from that entry to an elevator that reaches the desired floor (if needed), and the best way to go to the desired place. Since these paths must be achieved

TABLE 5.2

Analysis of Robot Orientation: Comparison Between Odometry and Computer Vision Measure by Mean Square Error (MSE), Standard Deviation, and Correlation With the Manual Measure.

		Odometry (o)	Vision (o)
Path 1	MSE	2.53	7.51
	Standard Deviation	1.46	5.88
	Correlation	0.937	−0.289
Path 2	MSE	2.80	7.64
	Standard Deviation	2.27	6.70
	Correlation	0.147	0.447
Path 3	MSE	2.48	7.60
	Standard Deviation	1.35	6.38
	Correlation	0.941	0.375
Path 4	MSE	2.95	7.63
	Standard Deviation	2.48	6.58
	Correlation	0.524	0.358
Path 5	MSE	2.59	5.29
	Standard Deviation	1.95	4.22
	Correlation	0.789	−0.508

by the wheelchair, they must not have stairs and doors that are difficult to open. This information is included in a set of XML building description files that describe the ways to access the building, the position of its entries (suitable to the wheelchair), and the map of each floor with the location of elevators, doors, and places of public access. They also define landmarks for wheelchair position calibration and optimum routes, free from physical barriers, from each landmark to all of its neighbors.

In the proposed architecture, a building to be visited is considered as having a ground floor, n floors, and k basements, defined by XML files with the formats described in following sections. Note that tags in XML files here described are named in Portuguese.

5.6.1 File Building.xml

This file (Figure 5.10) defines the number of floors and basements of the building, the position in UTM coordinates of the map of access to it, the

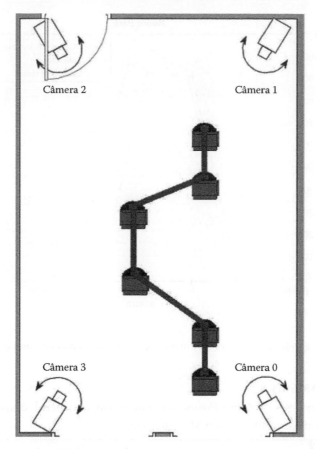

FIGURE 5.8
Curved path performed by the robot.

location and orientation of the ground floor on the map of access, and
the limits of the ground floor map in order to establish its initial scale
on the wheelchair computer screen. In this example the coordinates
are given in centimeters. The file also defines the existing elevators
and their connectivity (which floors can be reached with them).

5.6.2 Files Floor.xml

These files define the maps of each floor with doors and floor position
calibration marks (landmarks) for paths to be made by the wheelchair.

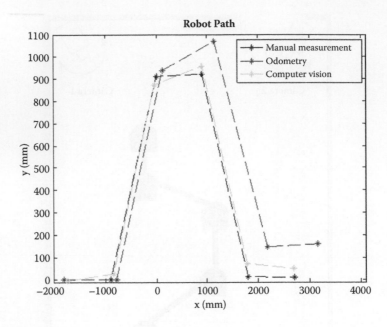

FIGURE 5.9
Experiment 2 graph—robot position by manual measurement, odometry, and computer vision.

TABLE 5.3

Analysis of Robot Position: Comparison Between Odometry and Computer Vision Measurement.

		Odometry (mm)	Vision (mm)
Path 1	MSE	180.7	41.38
	Standard Deviation	143.8	24.28
	Correlation	0.9967	0.9996
Path 2	MSE	172.0	51.02
	Standard Deviation	130.7	31.32
	Correlation	0.9982	0.9992
Path 3	MSE	203.9	39.64
	Standard Deviation	146.8	22.92
	Correlation	0.9976	0.9997
Path 4	MSE	166.9	40.48
	Standard Deviation	118.2	21.65
	Correlation	0.9987	0.9997
Path 5	MSE	187.5	37.15
	Standard Deviation	142.5	21.75
	Correlation	0.9981	0.9997

TABLE 5.4

Analysis of Robot Orientation: Comparison Between Odometry and Computer Vision Measurement.

		Odometry (mm)	Vision (mm)
Path 1	MSE	3.83	4.31
	Standard Deviation	3.01	2.59
	Correlation	0.995	0.996
Path 2	MSE	3.65	5.05
	Standard Deviation	2.73	4.13
	Correlation	0.993	0.992
Path 3	MSE	3.61	4.45
	Standard Deviation	2.66	3.31
	Correlation	0.991	0.992
Path 4	MSE	3.44	5.34
	Standard Deviation	2.59	3.54
	Correlation	0.999	0.992
Path 5	MSE	3.87	4.58
	Standard Deviation	3.08	2.69
	Correlation	0.995	0.996

```
<building name="Escuela Politécnica Superior">
  <floor number="3">
    <sector name="OESTEP3">
      <contour>
        <line  x_or="0" y_or="0" x_des="29,34" y_des="0" />
        <door  x_or="29,34" y_or="0" x_des="32,09" y_des="0" type="0"/>
        <line  x_or="32,09" y_or="0" x_des="41,76" y_des="0"/>
        <arc   x_or="41,76" y_or="0" x_des="63,75" y_des="21,99" r_x="67,9"
        <line  x_or="63,75" y_or="21,99" x_des="63,75" y_des="31,70"/>
        <door  x_or="63,75" y_or="31,70" x_des="63,75" y_des="34,49" type="0"/>
        <line  x_or="63,75" y_or="34,49" x_des="63,75" y_des="63,74"/>
        <line  x_or="63,75" y_or="63,74" x_des="37,47" y_des="63,74"/>
        <line  x_or="37,47" y_or="63,74" x_des="37,47" y_des="34,43"/>
        <line  x_or="37,47" y_or="34,43" x_des="29,31" y_des="26,28"/>
        <line  x_or="29,31" y_or="26,28" x_des="0" y_des="26,28"/>
        <line  x_or="0" y_or="26,28" x_des="0" y_des="0"/>
      </contour>
      <room name="F31" type="laboratory">
        <line  x_or="4,29" y_or="1,69" x_des="11,32" y_des="1,69" />
        <line  x_or="11,32" y_or="1,69" x_des="11,32" y_des="4,89" />
        <door  x_or="11,32" y_or="4,89" x_des="11,32" y_des="6,39" type="0" />
        <line  x_or="11,32" y_or="6,39" x_des="11,32" y_des="9,59" />
        <line  x_or="11,32" y_or="9,59" x_des="4,29" y_des="9,59"/>
        <line  x_or="4,29" y_or="9,59" x_des="4,29" y_des="1,69" />
      </room>
      ...
      ...

    </sector>
  </floor>
</building>
```

FIGURE 5.10
XML file with the basic building parameters.

```
1    <?xml version='1.0' encoding='utf-8'?>
2    <Andar>
3        <Rectangle X='3774' Y='255' Width='2333' Height='2380' Color='-1' />
4            : : :
5        <Rectangle X='7106' Y='255' Width='2584' Height='2380' Color='-1' />
6        <Line X1='2975' X1='13430' X2='340' Y2='13430' />
7            : : :
8        <Line X1='2975' X1='11883' X2='2975' Y2='13430' />
9        <Ellipse X='4148' Y='4216' Width='3202' Height='3236' Color='-1' />
10           : : :
11       <Ellipse X='1207' Y='1326' Width='714' Height='714' Color='-1' />
12       <Polygon NVertices='5' X0='9197' Y0='3383' X1='9435' Y1='3383' X2='9843'
13           Y2='3757' X3='9231' Y3='4333' X4='8772' Y4='3961' Color='-1' />
14       <Porta Name='PORTA1' X1='4803' Y1='11256' X2='4803' Y2='11427' />
15           : : :
16       <Porta Name='PORTA2' X1='4799' Y1='12036' X2='4799' Y2='12204' />
17       <Landmark Name='CIR24' Tipo='Circulacao' X1='6632' Y1='9247' X2='6832'
18           Y2='9447' Xo1='6732' Yo1='9447' Xo2='6732' Yo2='9247' />
19       <Landmark Name='ENT01' Tipo='Acesso' X1='463' Y1='6793' X2='663'
20           Y2='6993' Xo1='663' Yo1='6893' Xo2='463' Yo2='6893' />
21           : : :
22       <Landmark Name='ELEV1' Tipo='Elevador' X1='3690' Y1='7011' X2='3690'
23           Y2='7211' Xo1='3890' Yo1='7111' Xo2='3690' Yo2='7111' />
24   </Andar>
```

FIGURE 5.11
Floor XML file describing the floor map.

If a building has *n* floors and *k* basements with possible locations to be visited by the wheelchair, a total of $(n + k + 2)$ files with this structure result: a file for each floor, and basement, a file for the ground floor and a file for the building access map. Figure 5.11 shows the main fields of the XML floor files.

In this figure, a first set of lines represents the scale vector map of the floor and may be defined by geometric figures like lines, rectangles, ellipses, and polygons; the floor's reference is always considered to be in the top left corner of the picture. Next lines encode doors in corridors and rooms of places to be visited in the building. The last lines of the file represent positions and orientations of the calibration points (landmarks) of floor paths; these landmarks can define different behaviors that are coded in a type field; there are landmarks of circulation, landmarks of access to the building, and landmarks of floor elevators.

5.6.3 InfoFloor.xml

For each XML floor file, there is another XML file with the accessibility information of that floor. Figure 5.12 shows the format of the fields of the accessibility information.

This file defines all building sectors in the floor and the rooms or locations of each one of the sectors that could be visited. For each one of the defined locations, there are one or more sources that are a close landmark that can have a path from it to those locations. For

```
 1   <?xml version="1.0" encoding="utf-8"?>
 2   <InfoRadar0>
 3     <Setor Name="DEPARTAMENTO 1">
 4       <Local Name="XEROX">
 5         <Origem Name="CIR07" Distancia="3116">
 6           <Trecho Name="Landmark" NameLandmark="CIR07" />
 7           : : :
 8           <Trecho Name="Rota" X1="8429" Y1="1816" X2="9270" Y2="1867" Angulo="0" />
 9         </Origem>
10         <Origem Name="CIR06" Distancia="3279">
11           <Trecho Name="Landmark" NameLandmark="CIR06" />
12           : : :
13           <Trecho Name="Rota" X1="8613" Y1="1715" X2="9226" Y2="1732" Angulo="0" />
14         </Origem>
15       </Local>
16       <Local Name="SECRETARIA">
17         <Origem Name="CORR1" Distancia="2977">
18           <Trecho Name="Porta" NamePorta="PORTA1" NameCorredor="CORR1" />
19         </Origem>
20       </Local>
21     </Setor>
22     <Rota Origem="CIR01" Destino="ENT01" Distancia="2843">
23       <Trecho Name="Rota" X1="3118" Y1="7330" X2="3118" Y2="6943" Angulo="0" />
24       <Trecho Name="Rota" X1="3118" Y1="6943" X2="663" Y3="6893" Angulo="0" />
25     </Rota>
26     <Rota Origem="ENT01" Destino="CIR01" Distancia="2843">
27       <Trecho Name="Rota" X1="663" Y1="6893" X2="3118" Y2="6943" Angulo="0" />
28       <Trecho Name="Rota" X1="3118" Y1="6943" X2="3118" Y2="7330" Angulo="0" />
29     </Rota>
30     <Rota Origem="CIR01" Destino="CIR02" Distancia="868">
31       <Trecho Name="Rota" X1="3118" Y1="7330" X2="3064" Y2="6471" Angulo="0" />
32     </Rota>
33     <Corredor Name="CORR1" Origem="CORR1" Destino="" X1="5834" Y1="18993" X2="5817"
34       Y2="12893" Angulo="0" />
35   </InfoRadar0>
```

FIGURE 5.12
XML file structure of the floor accessibility information.

each source, a path connecting the landmark to the concerned place is defined. In Figure 5.12, a first set of lines, limited by "Setor" tag, shows the structure of definition of these rooms and paths in the XML file. The path from a landmark to a room can be defined as a sequence of straight lines or as a door associated with a corridor. Then, lines delimited with "Rota" tag show the fields of definition of the routes linking the landmarks with their neighbors. These routes are outlined following the best obstacle-free path for the wheelchair. Its length should not be very long, allowing the path-position control to be performed using the signals coming from the wheelchair odometry.

The final lines of Figure 5.12 show an example of the corridor definition on a floor ("Corredor" tag). The corridor is defined by a landmark and a line segment or two landmarks and a line segment (an existing route) linking the two landmarks. With the definition of doors associated with these corridors, the path of a landmark to the door can be generated automatically by the intersection of two straight lines.

Figure 5.13 shows a diagram of the accessibility information structure described in the defined XML files. Places of interest are stored as sectors. Each sector can have multiple locations and each location can be accessed by a number of sources, which are marks of navigation, represented by circles in Figure 5.13. The lines connecting the circles represent the routes defined between landmarks and their neighbors. The lines connecting the sources to the locations are paths to reach the location from the source.

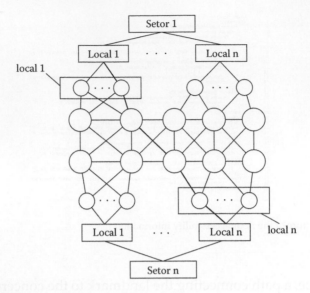

FIGURE 5.13
Sector, locations, and landmark tree for path planning.

The algorithm to plan the best route to go to another location takes into account the lower length path, using a variation of the Dijkstra algorithm [11] from all the existing routes in the XML file. All possible routes, using all possible sources, are analyzed, and the shortest path is chosen as the optimal one. If the destination is on the same floor where the wheelchair is, a direct path is found. If the destination is on another floor, the route is split first to get to the closest elevator that goes to both floors and then out of the elevator to the destination on the other floor, reaching the desired location. Once the route has been defined, the control program commands the wheelchair to follow a set of straight and circular paths in each part of the route. Wheelchair relative position is determined integrating encoder pulses (dead reckoning) between calibration landmarks. When the wheelchair reaches a landmark, absolute position and orientation information can be retrieved from it [7]. This information is used to correct dead-reckoning estimations.

Autonomous navigation can be overridden at any time by user actions by the laser sensor installed onboard the wheelchair. In case of a change in the existing routes, either by a placement of a fixed

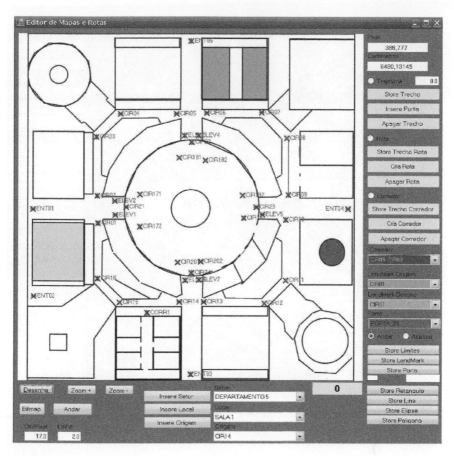

FIGURE 5.14
Screenshot of the accessibility information XML files editor. See color insert.

obstacle in the way, such as a kiosk in a mall, or a defective elevator or automatic door, building administrators must edit the affected route and send this modification to the server in a new XML file containing the change.

Figure 5.14 shows a screenshot of the developed accessibility information XML files editor. This tool allows the creation of vector maps for each of the building floors and the accessibility information (sectors, locations, sources, routes, and paths between locations and sources) for route and path planning.

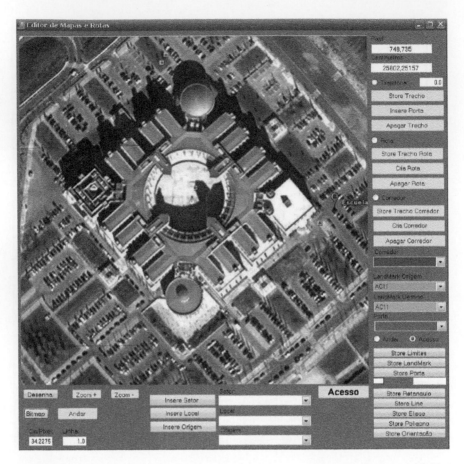

FIGURE 5.15
Edition of the building geographic position information screen. See color insert.

5.7 Sample

Figure 5.15 shows a picture of a georeferenced map of the Polytechnic School building of the University of Alcala (Spain). This building was used as an example for the creation of XML maps in the editor and to make the geographic position of the ground floor and the building access, along with their entries, accessible to the wheelchair.

Figure 5.16 shows the screen of the navigation setup program onboard the wheelchair. In the case shown in this figure, the user has

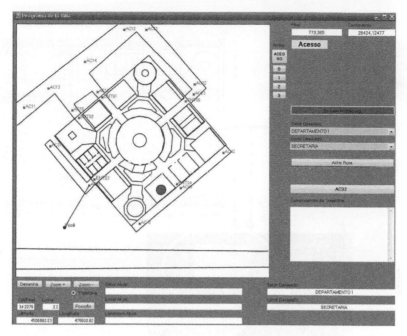

FIGURE 5.16
User position from the closest access entry to the building.

selected the Polytechnic School building. Once the accessibility information from the XML files is fetched, the screen of the geographic positioning of the ground floor will be available, along with the current position of the wheelchair and the building access nearest to the wheelchair. Thus, the desired location has been chosen, and the path planning has been done.

Figure 5.17 shows the path from entry 03 to the corresponding desired location, passing through each one of the existing landmarks for calibration. In this screen of the control program the user can navigate, selecting in the combo boxes the desired sector and location, using the mouse. If the user knows the desired locations directly on the map, they can be chosen directly using any of the modalities. This screen also allows the change of the building floor to perform the navigation between places in different floors.

The wheelchair control program makes the autonomous navigation from a point to the desired destination using each line segment and each landmark in the generated path shown in Figure 5.17. Figure 5.18 shows the wheelchair navigating in the building.

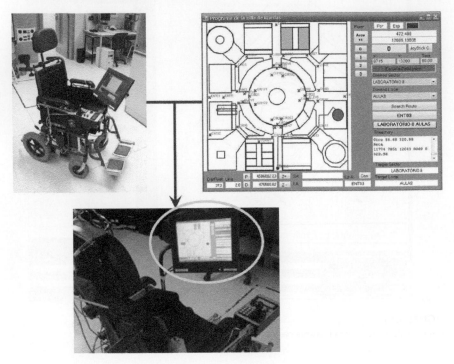

FIGURE 5.17
Path generated from entry 03 to the desired location.

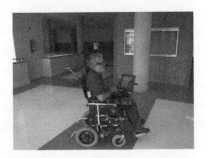

FIGURE 5.18
Wheelchair navigating in the building.

References

[1] D Ding, B Parmanto, H A Karimi, D Roongpiboonsopit, G Pramana, T Conahan, P Kasemsuppakorn, *Design considerations for a personalized wheelchair navigation system*. International Conference of the Engineering in Medicine and Biology Society, pp. 4790–4793, 2007.

[2] M Kurihara, H Nonaka, T Yoshikawa, *Use of highly accurate GPS in network-based barrier-free street map creation system*. International Conference on Systems, Man and Cybernetics, Vol. 2, pp. 1169–1173, 2004.

[3] O Matsumoto, K Komoriya, T Hatase, H Nishimura, H Tsutomu, N Hideki, *Autonomous traveling control of the TAO intelligent wheelchair*. International Conference on Intelligent Robots and Systems, Vol. 2, pp. 4322–4327, 2006.

[4] W Yi-Hui, L Bing-Yuh, C Heng-Yin, O Yao, L Jin-shin, K Te-Son, C Fok-Ching, *The development of M3S-based GPS navchair and telemonitor system*. International Conference of the Engineering in Medicine and Biology Society, Vol. 2, pp. 4052–4055, 2005.

[5] J C Garcia, M Marrón, M Mazo, J Ureña, *Positioning and localization system for autonomous wheelchairs*. Annual Conference of the Industrial Electronics Society, Vol. 2, pp. 1555–1560, 2002.

[6] P Jae-Han, B Seung-Ho, B Moon-Hong, *An intelligent navigation method for services robots in the smart environment*. International Conference on Control, Automation and Systems, pp. 494–497, 2007.

[7] M Marrón, J C García, *Sistema de navegación autónoma en entornos interiores estructurados*. TELEC'02 International Conference, pp. 1–4, 2002.

[8] H Chuan-heng, L Ming-long, S Yuan-Chung, L Feipei, *A design of small-area automatic wheelchair*. International Conference on Networking, Sensing and Control, Vol. 2, pp. 1341–1345, 2004.

[9] I Fernández, M Mazo, J Lázaro, D Pizarro, E Santiso, P Martín, C Losada, *Guidance of a mobile robot using an array of static cameras located in the environment*. Auton Robot, Vol. 23, pp. 305–324, 2007.

[10] E Aitenbichler, M Muhlhauser, *An IR local positioning system for smart items and devices*. 23rd International Conference on Distributed Computing Systems Workshops, pp. 334–339, 2003.

[11] E W Dijkstra, *A note on two problems in conexion with graphs*. Numer Math, pp. 269–271, 1959.

6

Walkers

Anselmo Frizera-Neto, Arlindo Elias-Neto, Carlos Cifuentes, Carlos
Valadão, Valmir Schneider-Junior, Camilo Díaz, and Teodiano Freire
Bastos-Filho
Universidade Federal do Espírito Santo, Brazil

Ricardo Carelli
Universidad Nacional de San Juan, Argentina

CONTENTS

6.1 Introduction

Mobility is one of the most important human faculties. It affects
not only the individual's locomotion capacity but also the ability to

perform certain tasks, affecting physiological and personal aspects and conditioning the conduct of an individual in his/her environment.

Different types of pathologies, such as poliomyelitis, spinal cord injuries, multiple sclerosis, and trauma, affect human mobility at different levels, causing partial or total loss of such faculties. In addition, it is known that mobility decreases gradually with age as a consequence of neurological, muscular, and/or osteoarticular deterioration.

An individual may need devices to replace, maintain, recover, and empower his/her locomotion capacities. The selection of an individual's mobility assistive device should be made according to the pathology and the degree of illness or physical disability of the individual.

Considering the several types of conditions that affect human mobility, it is necessary to take into account the level of motor impairment during the selection of a technical aid. In the case of total incapacity of mobility, standing, and locomotion, alternative solutions such as wheelchairs or special vehicles (e.g., scooters) should be addressed. As mentioned in previous chapters, robotic wheelchairs have been an intense focus of research during the past two decades. Autonomous and assisted navigation using several types of human–machine interfaces (HMIs) have been proposed in order to restore locomotion in many rehabilitation scenarios. Such research has created a wide discussion in the scientific community and formed a doctrine body, the Autonomous Robotic Wheelchairs (ARW). Examples and applications of ARW are presented in this book (Chapters 3, 4, and 5) and, therefore, will not be further discussed in this chapter.

However, it is known that the continuous use of wheelchairs can cause problems such as joint stiffness, skin ulcerations, deformities in the spinal cord, and physiological dysfunctions, all related to remaining in a seated position for long periods of time. For such reasons, the use of some alternative devices should be avoided if the user prefers certain locomotion capabilities preserved. People with disabilities are usually encouraged by the rehabilitation staff to use augmentative devices that aim to empower the user's natural means of locomotion, the lower limbs, taking advantage of the remaining motor capabilities. This second group of rehabilitation devices can be classified into wearable—orthoses and prostheses—or external devices—canes, crutches, and walkers. Currently, augmentative devices are also a great focus of research and advanced/robotic solutions are easily found in the literature.

6.2 Devices for Mobility

Mobility problems constantly challenge the ability of physical therapists to restore patients' activities of daily living and quality of life [1]. Immobilization can elicit profound effects in the musculoskeletal system, significantly changing histology and normal mechanics of the tissues involved, which reflects in poor postural control, muscle weakness, and altered gait biomechanics [2] [3] [4]. On the other hand, elderly persons with neurodegenerative conditions [5] and patients with spinal cord injury [2] or submitted to lower-limb orthopedic surgery are among the people with an increased risk of developing immobilization-related dysfunctions [1].

Efficient rehabilitation strategies rely on early mobilization procedures and training to prevent the deleterious effects of immobilization [1] [3]. In the case of orthopedic patients, physical therapy begins while patients are still in the infirmary, encouraging active joint movements and deambulation as soon as possible [6]. Elderly people benefit greatly from a rehabilitation program since it can prevent functional decline associated with aging, which leads to progressive disability and related morbidity and mortality [7] [8].

A key point in rehabilitation is the treatment progression. Here, physical therapists stimulate the patient to perform more challenging tasks when their functional status reaches predetermined levels during the course of treatment [1]. In order to adequately progress through the rehabilitation program, the use of assistive devices, such as canes or walkers, is helpful and, in some cases, imperative.

External devices, such as crutches, canes, and walkers, are very commonly found in daily life. There are many variations of such devices according to the user's necessities, such as the patient's cognitive function, judgment, vision, vestibular function, upper body strength, physical endurance, and living environment [5]. Nevertheless, advanced or robotic versions of such devices are not as current as wheelchairs. Usually, robotic canes are more focused on assisting the user's navigation than on offering physical support.

Walkers improve balance by increasing the patient's base of support, enhancing lateral stability, and supporting the patient's weight. There are many types of walkers, considering their constitutive materials, accessories, sizes, and structural configurations. Nevertheless, an important aspect that classifies conventional walkers is the ground contact configuration. There are devices that only have legs, others with legs and wheels, and, finally, three- or four-wheeled walkers [9]. Other studies present a complementary classification of standard walkers in three major types [10]. Standard walking frames or Zimmer frames are designed to provide a larger base of support to a person with lower-limb weakness.

Rollators are walking frames with wheels attached and there are many different configurations of the base. Rollators are used where balance is the major problem rather than a need for weight bearing. They are also used where upper limb strength is not sufficient to lift the walking frame on a regular basis. This device should be used if the patient requires a larger base of support and does not rely on the walker to bear weight. If a patient applies full body weight on the device, it could roll away, resulting in a fall [5].

Reciprocal frames are devices similar to the standard frames except that the frame is hinged on either side, allowing the sides of the frame to be moved alternately. They are designed to accommodate a normal walking pattern with opposite arm and leg moving together. They are also used in domestic homes where space is confined.

In addition to the three types of walkers previously presented, there are the front-wheeled walkers. These devices are an intermediary device between Zimmer frames and rollators. Wheels permit the patient to maintain a more normal gait pattern than they would with a standard walker, but they also decrease stability. van Hook et al. present a detailed study concerning the different types of walkers and their application to certain gait disorders [5].

Despite enhanced support and utility for weight bearing, walkers also have disadvantages. These include difficulty maneuvering the device through doorways and congested areas, reduction in normal arm swing, and poor posture with abnormal flexion of the back while walking. In general, walkers should not be used on stairs [5]. Conventional walkers also present problems related to the pushing energy required to move the device, lack of stability and brake control (especially in rollators), and the possibility of collision with obstacles.

In this context, to solve those issues, robotic or smart walkers are a major focus of research in many groups. Such devices aim at potentiating the user's residual mobility capacities by means of advanced human–machine interfaces and controlled guidance. Smart walkers play an important role in treatment planning and progression since they present several features that can be explored for rehabilitation purposes by health professionals. Several systems are discussed in literature, each one presenting different combinations of features that focus mainly on attending to the needs of the elderly population [11], while their potential role in physical therapy programs remains largely unexplored.

6.3 Potential Clinical Applications and Feature-Based Classification of Smart Walkers

Smart walkers provide assistance to the user at different levels, depending on the user's needs. A functional classification of such devices is presented.

6.3.1 Physical Stability and Motion Support

There are two classic types of physical stability and motion support that can be provided by smart walkers: active and passive [9] [12]. In passive devices, the user has to provide the total amount of pushing energy to the device. The system tends to be lighter and simpler to assemble. It can also be equipped with several security mechanisms, like obstacle avoidance and special braking capabilities [13] [14]. When using this type of walker, users must have adequate postural control and walking ability [15], making the device suitable for later stages of rehabilitation programs and mostly for functional compensation.

Active walkers, on the other hand, are capable of automatic propelling power and navigation, providing better control of overall movement characteristics, like speed, direction, and slope negotiation [9] [12]. This is translated into a much safer device that can be indicated for patients in the early stages of rehabilitation or presenting a high degree of frailty and decreased motor functions in chronic stages. However, the construction of this type of walker is more complex than a passive system [15], and the need for extra electronic components may be reflected in higher costs.

Hybrid systems are also described in the literature, where both types of control can coexist in the device [12] [17]. This feature is especially interesting for rehabilitation purposes, since training programs can be progressed from early stages, with more active control features required, to advanced programs, where passive control can be used to enhance proprioception and walking abilities of the patient.

Besides assisting in the user's locomotion, some smart walker systems are also capable of assisting other functional tasks like sit-to-stand or stand-to-sit transfers [22] [23] [24]. The versatility of these multifunctional systems can have a positive impact in several clinical scenarios where upright postural training or stimulation are needed, such as patients in the immediate postoperative phase of lower-limb orthopedic surgery or the elderly with poor postural control and lower-limb weakness, and patients presenting pathological gait conditions like stroke or multiple sclerosis.

Several models of smart walkers have force sensors embedded in the handles of the device [20]. This is important to detect the user's intent to move, and it enhances the cognitive human–machine interaction. Force signals are converted into guidance commands through filtering and classification strategies [19]. In addition, involuntary force interaction components do not generate motor commands, contributing actively to an increase in safety during assisted locomotion.

An innovative forearm support was addressed in the Simbiosis project, and was also used to detect force interaction patterns during motion tasks and to identify the user's intent of movement [9] [19]. The detection of force patterns, both in handles or alternative supports, can also be used to identify altered gait patterns that can be corrected by a feedback intervention by the physical therapist.

6.3.2 Navigation and Localization Components

Navigation systems are a constant addition in several smart walkers. The main objective is to provide safer locomotion to the user, since the sensors embedded in the walker are able to detect obstacles and, in some cases, automatically avoid them through an alternate route or, at least, notify the user about their presence. This feature is of special interest for people with severe visual disturbances [18] and may act in conjunction with active systems to drive the user safely through an environment.

This function can be accomplished by previous knowledge of the environment's map [18] or by real-time obstacle detection and negotiation [16]. The first mode is suitable for closed environments, such as homes or clinical scenarios. The latter mode is indicated in open or multiple environments, being suitable for patients with a more active lifestyle, using the device daily for functional compensation. In either way, these features may give more confidence to the patient in the early stages of rehabilitation programs, and gait training can be safely done in either ambulatory or hospital settings, or even at home. The devices can also communicate with the user via visual or voice feedback, informing the user of the presence of obstacles and giving direction options [12] [18].

Autonomous localization features are relevant for patients with cognitive disturbance, sensory degradation, and loss of memory, which are associated with neurodegenerative diseases such as Alzheimer's or Parkinson's. GPS locators can be installed in smart walkers in order to keep track of the patient in a particular environment or outside [9].

Modern systems are also able to interact with specific sensors in the environment, providing the patient with direction options and localization via visual feedback [21].

6.3.3 Biomechanical and Bioelectrical Monitoring

Besides movement and navigation assistance, smart walkers present monitoring features that are of significant relevance for rehabilitation programs. Recent studies investigating gait parameters have shown the potential and versatility of this type of assistive device in treatment planning and progression. This feature also adds the possibility of out-of-the-clinic monitoring.

In a clinical setting, several gait parameters can be monitored by therapists in a treatment session using smart walkers, including speed of movement, total distance walked, characteristics of gait phases, total amount of force/torque exerted in the handles during gait tasks, movement acceleration/deceleration, stride length, and several others [25] [26] [27] [28] [29].

The detection of dysfunctional gait patterns, presented during training sessions with smart walkers, can provide crucial information that can be used by the clinician to enhance the overall treatment program and progression, which can reflect in increased precision and quality of the intervention.

In addition to biomechanical and bioelectrical data analysis, the monitoring of other physiological signals through smart walkers is also possible and can be used to keep track of associated comorbidities of the user. The PAMM system, developed by MIT, was the first to present an embedded electrocardiogram monitoring system [30]. Modern walkers are also able to monitor blood oxygenation through a photoplethysmography sensor located in the handles of the device [26] [27].

All this information can be used to record a medical and/or functional history of the user and can also be sent via a remote terminal to the professional staff responsible for the rehabilitation program [9] [28] [30].

6.3.4 Safety Measures

Safety is a major concern of smart walker systems, since the user must rely on the support provided by the device to perform the necessary tasks of rehabilitation programs or activities of daily living.

Several systems present a variety of strategies to prevent falls and to help stabilize the user's gait pattern. The main features associated with this function are braking, irregular movement detection, gravity compensation, and user–walker distance monitoring.

Emergency braking strategies are often associated with obstacles and stair detection, acting in conjunction with navigation components [14] [15] [16]. Gravity compensation is another feature that makes use of intelligent navigation, allowing the recognition and proper negotiation of terrain irregularities, such as slopes [15].

Rapid irregular or jerky movements are indicative of postural imbalance and can be detected by force sensors in either handles or forearm support [9], braking the device to provide enough support for postural recovery [19].

A remarkable feature of some systems is related to the placement of rear sensors in the device. The objective is to constantly monitor the distance between the user and the walker. An increase of this distance is detected by the rear sensor and emergency braking is performed, allowing the user to reestablish the correct, and safer, distance [14].

A recent model presented an innovative step-by-step technology that enabled the walker to keep the same speed of the user in a more dynamic way, by monitoring the user's footsteps [12].

Braking the device is also important to provide support for sit-to-stand and stand-to-sit assistance, avoiding slipping or undesired movement of the walker that could increase the chance of falls [15] [18].

TABLE 6.1

Feature-Based Classification of Smart Walkers

Classification	Related function	Features
Physical stability and motion support	Propelling power	Passive, active, and hybrid systems
	Motor task assistance	Walking and multitask assistance
	Movement intent detection	Handle force sensors
Navigation and localization components	Intelligent navigation	Installed maps Obstacle avoidance Environment interaction Embedded GPS
	Localization assistance	Visual and voice feedback Automatic return to selected location
Biomechanical and bioelectrical monitoring	Functional monitoring	Gait and/or specific motor task parameters
	Physiological monitoring	Biosignal monitoring
Safety measures	Fall prevention	Braking Involuntary movement detection User-device distance Gravity compensation

Table 6.1 summarizes all the discussed functions and characteristics of smart walkers.

6.4 UFES Smart Walker

6.4.1 System Description and Concepts

Based on the aforementioned features, summarized in Table 6.1, a smart walker suitable for both physical therapy practice and domicile use in functional compensation was developed in UFES/Brazil. The system has two main users: the patient and the clinician assisting in the rehabilitation program.

The UFES Smart Walker (Figure 6.1) is a rollator equipped with two drive-wheels and one free-wheel. To perform the rehabilitation and functional compensation strategies, the device integrates a PC/104+ embedded computer responsible for the high-level controller, a signal acquisition board for interfacing with a series of sensors, and a network board to allow programming mobility strategies and saving the experiment data for further analysis. The low-level controller is performed by a separate custom board that ensures the correct functioning

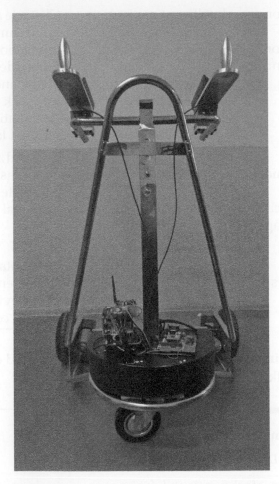

FIGURE 6.1
Different views of UFES Smart Walker. *(Continued)*

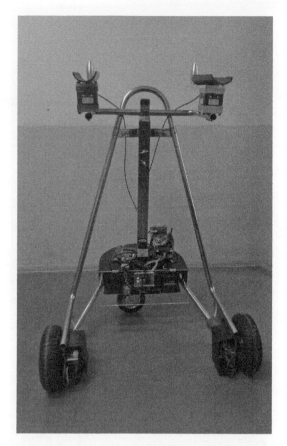

FIGURE 6.1
(Continued). Different views of UFES Smart Walker. *(Continued)*

of each motorized wheel and integrates safety functions to protect the user and the electronic components in case of failure. A closed-loop proportional-integral-derivative (PID) controller is installed and two optical encoders provide odometry information.

Two force sensors (model MTA400 from Futek) acquire the interaction forces applied by the users in the force support platforms. A laser sensor (model URG-04LX from Hokuyo) and custom hardware measure and track in real time the user's feet. Gait patterns and muscular activation can be acquired and fed into the high-level control system for a personalized control strategy based on the current state of the patient. This is done by means of a wireless motion-capture system based on inertial measurement units developed by the research group. Figure 6.2

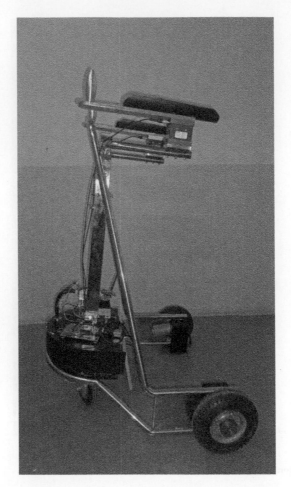

FIGURE 6.1
(Continued). Different views of UFES Smart Walker.

shows a complete view of the developed system indicating the most important components.

The walker uses a high-level inverse kinematics controller to compensate for the nonlinearities of the system, thus obtaining a linear closed-loop system. Using this approach, it is possible to control two important variables: the distance between the user and the device (d), and the angle between the user instantaneous speed and the user–laser axis (φ). Figure 6.3 illustrates these variables and the kinematic model used in the control algorithm. All the variables necessary for the

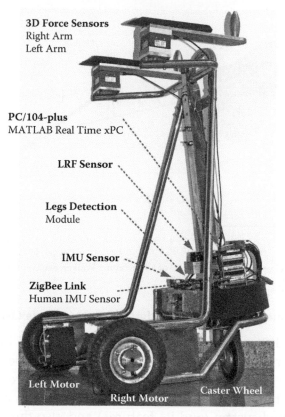

3D Force Sensors
Right Arm
Left Arm

PC/104-plus
MATLAB Real Time xPC

LRF Sensor

Legs Detection
Module

IMU Sensor

ZigBee Link
Human IMU Sensor

Left Motor

Right Motor

Caster Wheel

FIGURE 6.2
Details of UFES Smart Walker. See color insert.

execution of the control strategy are obtained using the sensor subsystems previously presented.

It is possible to express the kinematic model of the walker–human system and estimate the variables needed by the control algorithm, which are provided by the laser sensor. Using the controller design based on inverse kinematics, the control actions can be expressed as

$$V_w = \cos\theta \left[-k_d\tilde{d} + V_h \cos\varphi\right] - d\sin\theta \left[-k_\varphi\varphi - \omega_h - \frac{V_h}{d}\sin\varphi\right]$$

$$\omega_w = -\frac{\sin\theta}{a}\left[-k_d\tilde{d} + V_h\cos\varphi\right] - \frac{d}{a}\cos\theta\left[-k_\varphi\varphi - \omega_h - \frac{V_h}{d}\sin\varphi\right]$$

The control errors, considering the positive control gains, will always converge to zero.

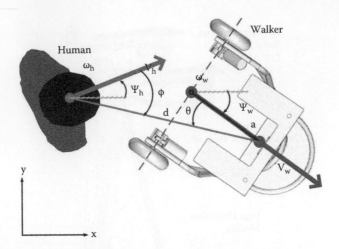

FIGURE 6.3
Kinematic model used for the controller of UFES Smart Walker. See color insert.

6.4.2 Experiments with Patients Suffering from Moderate Osteoarthritis

The many different smart walker models described in the literature present numerous features and resources that can be used for rehabilitation or functional compensation purposes. However, most of the published studies to date are concerned mainly with a description of the developed system (and its features) and also the potential benefits for the users. Thus, there is a gap in the literature in regard to real clinical applications involving such devices, especially on the measurement of their impact over gait biomechanical parameters of subjects with musculoskeletal or neurological impairments.

This section presents results of experiments about the kinematic behavior of the knee of subjects with moderate osteoarthritis (OA). The main objective is to assess the angular motion of the affected knee in the sagittal plane during normal and assisted ambulation with the UFES walker.

6.4.3 Sample

The study sample was composed of women with bilateral moderate knee OA, over 55 years old, able to walk without assistance for at least 25 meters, not having done any rehabilitation treatment for at least two months, and without analgesic medication in the last week. The diagnosis of knee OA was established based on the clinical and

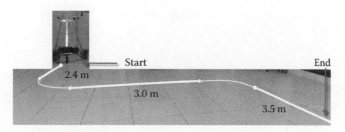

FIGURE 6.4
Path used during the experiments with the UFES Smart Walker.

radiographic criteria of the American College of Rheumatology, which present 91 percent sensitivity and 86 percent diagnostic specificity [31] [32]. Figure 6.4 shows the path used during the trials, and Figure 6.5 shows some volunteers conducting the experiments.

Sample size was calculated based on the mean paired difference of parameters with two-tailed significance, effect size adjusted for 0.7 (Cohen's criteria), 80 percent of statistical power, and an alpha of 0.05. The results indicated a minimum sample size of 15 subjects, which is compatible with the samples of other studies of gait biomechanics of elderly individuals with knee OA.

The exclusion criteria used during the selection process included recent trauma; history of previous surgery of the lower limbs, pelvis, or lumbar spine; neuromuscular diseases and other pathological forms of arthritis; chronic cardiovascular disease; orthopedic disorders of the upper limbs that prevented load support by the forearms; and unilateral knee OA. At the end of the selection process, 15 women met the inclusion criteria and volunteered to participate in the experimental procedure. The classification of subjects with moderate OA was based on the radiological criteria of Kellgren-Lawrence grade 2 or 3, physical examination, and no indication of total knee arthroplasty [36] [33]. According to [33], such criteria result in appropriate division between subjects with moderate and severe OA. Additional clinical information included functional assessment through the Western Ontario and McMasters University Questionnaire (WOMAC), demographic data, and perceived pain using a visual analogue scale (VAS).

All participants gave informed consent prior to the beginning of the tests. The experimental protocol was approved by the local ethics committee of UFES/Brazil.

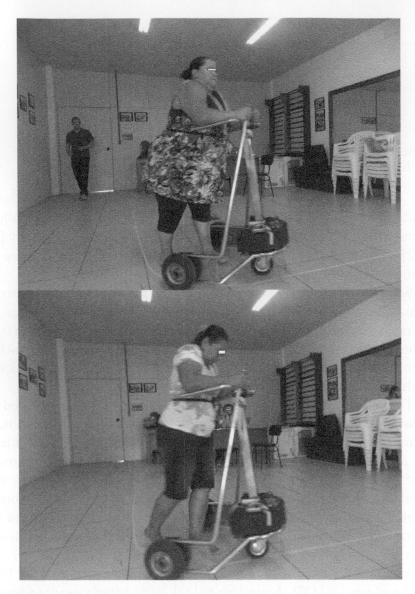

FIGURE 6.5
Volunteers conducting the experiments. *(Continued)*

6.4.4 Experimental Procedure

The gait analysis experiment was conducted at a public rehabilitation center (CREFES/Brazil), in a room dedicated to group rehabilitation activities whose dimensions were adequate for the testing.

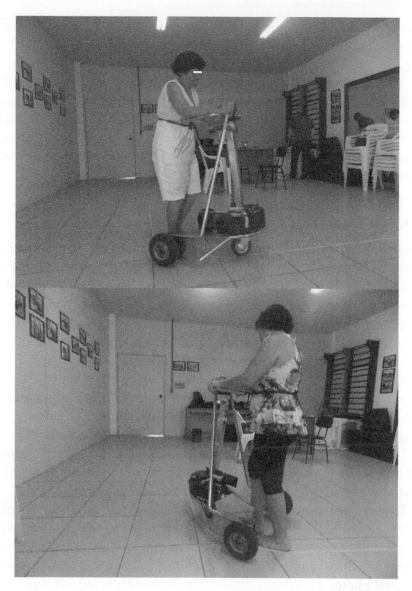

FIGURE 6.5
(Continued). Volunteers conducting the experiments.

The participants completed the demographic and clinical forms before the beginning of the tests. All subjects were instructed about the purposes of the experiment, but no pretest familiarization with the walker was conducted, with the objective of evaluating the ease of use of the device in a real functional compensation scenario. The kinematic parameters of the knee joint were acquired with two inertial measurement units (IMUs), positioned at the anterior aspect of the thigh and leg.

After calibration of the sensors, the patients were positioned at the beginning of the test walkway and asked to walk a straight line along the path. Each subject was asked to perform five free walking tests and five tests of walking assisted with the UFES Smart Walker. However, due to pain during walking, some patients underwent fewer repetitions, but not less than three in each test.

6.4.5 Data Acquisition and Extraction of the Kinematic Variables

The use of inertial sensors in studies regarding kinematic gait parameters is still recent in the literature, and standardized protocols for their use in clinical applications (especially involving knee assessment) are scarce. However, recent studies have shown that the use of such devices is more suited to routine clinical practice and was associated with lower operating costs when compared to traditional optoelectronic devices.

The sagittal knee angles were extracted by using two wearable IMUs with wireless communication (ZigBee). Each sensor sends tridimensional data of acceleration, angular velocity, and orientation (roll, pitch, yaw) through the ZigBee network to another sensor that acts as the coordinator. The signals are acquired at a sampling frequency of 50 Hz.

The portability of the IMUs was also a factor considered in the selection of the measurement device, because it allows the walker to be tested in different environments, outside the laboratory setting.

To measure the angular displacement of the knee in the sagittal plane, the angles (pitch) of the thigh and leg were subtracted. Figure 6.6 shows the angles of each sensor and the result of subtraction, generating the characteristic waveform of the kinematic behavior of the knee in the sagittal plane.

The discreet kinematic parameters evaluated in this study were based on previous research by [35]. However, the IMUs alone were not able to estimate the precise toe-off instant, and the beginning of the swing phase wasn't computed. The extraction of the remaining parameters was performed manually on the plots generated by the MATLAB platform after processing. The first and last cycles of each test series were excluded and only the intermediate cycles were considered for analysis (Figure 6.7).

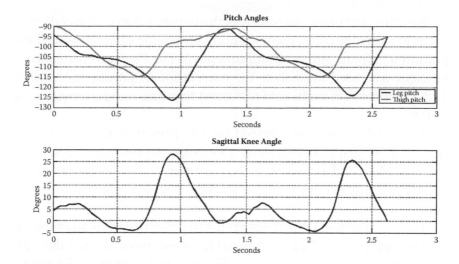

FIGURE 6.6
Kinematic behavior of the knee angle in the sagittal plane.

6.4.6 Statistical Analysis

For the statistical analysis, the null hypothesis was defined as the absence of significant paired differences between the correspondent normal and walker-assisted parameters.

Initially, descriptive statistics were presented for each parameter of interest. In the second phase, all datasets were analyzed by the Shapiro-Wilk test to assess the distribution patterns. Based on such results, the pairs of variables with Gaussian distribution were compared using the Student's paired samples t-test, whereas nonparametric variables were compared using the Wilcoxon signed rank test.

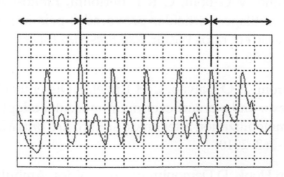

FIGURE 6.7
Cycles considered for kinematic analysis.

The third part of the analysis was the construction of correlation matrices to study the relationships among kinematic variables and clinical parameters (pain, stiffness, and function). The Pearson correlation coefficient was used to analyze the correlation of parametric variables and the Spearman coefficient was used to assess nonparametric counterparts.

The signals were also assessed for the presence of excessive noise (from sensor displacement during locomotion) that could corrupt the interpretation and extraction of the parameters. A set of parameters for each test condition (normal and walker assisted) is stored for further statistical analysis.

The results showed that the overall gait pattern of the walker-assisted ambulation was marked by reduced knee extension during the stance phase, reduced flexion during oscillation, and consequently, reduced joint excursion in the sagittal plane when compared with a previous walker-assisted experiment with normal subjects [34].

References

[1] R Cantu, *Soft Tissue Healing Considerations after Surgery*. Mosby, St. Louis, 2001, pp. 2–11.

[2] W A Rocha, G A Gobbi, V F Araujo, C H Santuzzi, B V Nogueira, W L Gonçalves, Muscle morphological changes in response to passive stretching in an animal model of prolonged immobilization of hind limb, *Rev Bras Med*, Vol. 16 (6), pp. 450–454, 2010.

[3] D Portinho, V G Boin, G R F Bertolini, Efeitos sobre o tecido ósseo e cartilagem articular provocados pela imobilização e remobilização em ratos Wistar, *Rev Bras Med Esporte*, Vol. 14 (5), pp. 408–411, 2008.

[4] B M Baroni, A Q Galvão, C H Ritzel, F Diefenthaeler, M A Vaz, Dorsiflexor and plantarflexor neuromuscular adaptations at two-week immobilization after ankle sprain, *Rev Bras Med*, Vol. 16 (5), pp. 358–362, 2010.

[5] F W van Hook, D Demonbreun, B D Weiss, Ambulatory devices for chronic gait disorders in the elderly, *Am Fam Physician*, Vol. 67 (8), pp. 1717–1724, 2003.

[6] G DeJong, C H. Hsieh, J Gassaway, S D Horn, R J Smout, K Putman, R James, M Brown, E M Newman, M P Foley, Characterizing rehabilitation services for patients with knee and hip replacement in skilled nursing facilities and inpatient rehabilitation facilities. *Arch Phys Med Rehab*, Vol. 90 (8), pp. 1269–1283, 2009.

[7] T Gill, D Baker, M Gottschalk, P Peduzzi, H Allore, P Vanness, A prehabilitation program for the prevention of functional decline: Effect on higher-level physical function, *Arch Phys Med Rehab*, Vol. 85 (7), pp. 1043–1049, 2004.

[8] M J Faber, R J Bosscher, M J Chin, A Paw, P C van Wieringen, Effects of exercise programs on falls and mobility in frail and pre-frail older adults: A multicenter randomized controlled trial. *Arch Phys Med Rehab*, Vol. 87 (7), pp. 885–896, 2006.

[9] A Frizera, R Ceres, J L Pons, A Abellanas, R Raya, *The smart walkers as geriatric assistive device. The SIMBIOSIS Purpose.* Proceedings of the 6th International Conference of the International Society for Gerontechnology, pp. 1–6, 2008.

[10] G Lacey, K Dawson-Howe, *Evaluation of robot mobility aid for the elderly blind.* Proceedings of the Fifth International Symposium on Intelligent Robotic Systems, pp. 1–7, 1997.

[11] P Rumeau, V Pasquiboutard, M Schaff, S Moulias, P Mederic, F Steenkeste, F. Piette, B Vellas, N Noury, V Dupourquet, *Techniques de la robotique: Application au développement de déambulateurs adaptés au handicap à la marche des personnes âgées.* NPG Neurologie—Psychiatrie—Gériatrie, vol. 5 (25), pp. 31–37, 2005.

[12] K T Yu, C P Lam, M F Chang, W H Mou, S H Tseng, L C Fu, *An interactive robotic walker for assisting elderly mobility in senior care unit.* Workshop on Advanced Robotics and Its Social Impacts, pp. 24–29, 2010.

[13] S MacNamara, G Lacey, *A smart walker for the frail visually impaired.* International Conference on Robotics and Automaton, Vol. 2, pp. 1354–1359, 2010.

[14] Y Hirata, A Muraki, K Kosuge, *Motion control of intelligent passive-type walker for fall-prevention function based on estimation of user state.*

International Conference on Robotics and Automation, pp. 3498–3503, 2006.

[15] Y Hirata, T Baba, K Kosuge, *Standing up and sitting down support using intelligent walker based on estimation of user states*. International Conference on Mechatronics and Automation, pp. 13–18, 2006.

[16] B Graf, *An adaptive guidance system for robotic walking aids*. J Comput Inf Technol, Vol. 1, pp. 109–120, 2008.

[17] A Morris, R Donamukkalat, A Steinfeldt, J Dunbarjacob, *A robotic walker that provides guidance*. International Conference on Robotics, pp. 25–30, 2003.

[18] D Rodriguez-Losada, F Matia, A Jimenez, G Lacey, *Guido, the robotic smart walker for the frail visually impaired*. International Conference on Domotics, Robotics and Remote Assistance for All, 2005.

[19] A Abellanas, A Frizera, R Ceres, R Raya, *Assessment of the laterality effects through forearm reaction forces in walker assisted gait*. Procedia Chemistry, Vol. 1 (1), pp. 1227–1230, 2009.

[20] P Mederic, F Plumet, P Bidaud, *Design of a walking-aid and sit to stand transfer assisting device for elderly people*. Symposium on Robot Design, Dynamics and Control, 2004.

[21] V Kulyukin, A Kutiyanawala, E LoPresti, J Matthews, R Simpson, *iWalker: Toward a rollator-mounted wayfinding system for the elderly*. International Conference on RFID, pp. 303–311, 2008.

[22] A J Rentschler, R A Cooper, B Blasch, M L Boninger, *Intelligent walkers for the elderly: Performance and safety testing of VA-PAMAID robotic walker*. J Rehab Res Dev, Vol. 40 (5), pp. 423–432, 2003.

[23] D Chugo, W Matsuoka, S Jia, K Takase, *A robotic walker with standing assistance*. International Conference on Information and Automation, pp. 452–457, 2008.

[24] D Chugo, T Asawa, T Kitamura, S Jia, K Takase, *A rehabilitation walker with standing and walking assistance*. International Conference on Intelligent Robots and Systems, 2008.

[25] C Zong, M Chetouani, A Tapus, *Automatic gait characterization for a mobility assistance system*. International Conference in Control, Automation, Robotics and Vision, pp. 473–478, 2010.

[26] A D C Chan, J R Green, *Smart rollator prototype*. International Workshop on Medical Measurements and Applications, pp. 97–100, 2008.

[27] M Alwan, G Wasson, P Sheth, A Ledoux, C Huang, *Passive derivation of basic walker-assisted gait characteristics from measured forces and moments*. International Conference of the IEEE EMBS, pp. 2691–2694, 2004.

[28] S Dubowsky, F Genot, S Godding, H Kozono, A Skwersky, *PAMM—a robotic aid to the elderly for mobility assistance and monitoring: A helping-hand for the elderly*. International Conference on Robotics and Automation, pp. 570–576, 2000.

[29] J Henry, *Gait monitoring for the elderly using a robotic walking aid*. Convention of Electrical and Electronics Engineers, pp. 392–394, 2010.

[30] H Y Spenko, S Dubowsky, *Robotic personal aids for mobility and monitoring for the elderly*. IEEE T Neur Sys Reh, Vol. 14 (3), pp. 344–351, 2006.

[31] R Altman, E Asch, D Bloch, *Development of criteria for the classification and reporting of osteoarthritis: classification of osteoarthritis of the knee*. Arthritis Rheum, Vol. 29 (8), pp. 1039–1049, 1986.

[32] Y Nagano, K Naito, Y Saho, *Association between in vivo knee kinematics during gait and the severity of knee osteoarthritis*. Knee, Vol. 19 (5), pp. 628–632, 2012.

[33] J L Astephen, K J Deluzio, G E Caldwell, M J Dunbar, C L Hubley-Kozey, *Gait and neuromuscular pattern changes are associated with differences in knee osteoarthritis severity levels*. J Biomech, Vol. 41 (4), pp. 868–876, 2008.

[34] A Frizera, A Elias, J Antonio, R Ceres, T F Bastos, *Characterization of spatio-temporal parameters of human gait assisted by a robotic walker*. International Conference on Biomedical Robotics and Biomechatronics, pp. 1087–1091, 2012.

[35] M G Benedetti, F Catani, A Leardini, E Pignotti, S Giannini, *Data management in gait analysis for clinical applications*. Clin Biomech, pp. 204–215, 1998.

[36] J A Zeni, J S Higginson, *Differences in gait parameters between healthy subjects and persons with moderate and severe knee osteoarthritis: a result of altered walking speed?* Clin Biomech, Vol. 24 (4), pp. 372–378, 2009.

7

Manipulation Technologies for Developing Cognitive Skills

Carlos Valadão, Jhon Sarmiento-Vela, Christiane Goulart, Javier Castillo,
and Teodiano Freire Bastos-Filho
Universidade Federal do Espírito Santo, Brazil

CONTENTS

7.1 Introduction

Learning in childhood is done by exploration, manipulation and discovery of the environment. The first two years of a child's life is the sensorial motor period [1]. During this stage of development, interaction with the environment is done through manipulation and body stimulus [2]. This means that children learn about their own bodies and the interaction of their own bodies with the environment by repetitive experiments and exploring the world around them through their senses [3].

This spatial object manipulation and environmental interaction are fundamental for the child's cognitive development. At the end of this sensorial-motor period, normal children should have the notion of space, position of objects inside the space and time, and some relation among them [3]. However, those children who have suffered neuromuscular disorders do not develop these skills. This impairs their ability to experience their own bodies and the world and delays growth compared with other children, which results in learning difficulties and their social isolation. This makes such children very dependent on their parents or caretakers to interact with the world [4], and this may restrict their cognitive and social development.

This inability of a child to explore his/her environment independently results in a lack of interest in exploration, and consequently such children become " helplessness learners" [6]. They see themselves as unable to do anything independently and usually adopt a passivity and lack of interest behavior toward the world in which they live.

To overcome these developmental difficulties of children who have impaired neuromotor skills, it is necessary that the children have a way to explore the world through alternative methods such as object manipulation [5]. This will help these children improve their self-esteem and expand their personal and social development, and prevent them from becoming " helplessness learners" [6].

Advancements in robotics and interactive simulation techniques have resulted in the development of Assistive technologies for Developing Cognitive Skills (ADCS) that can be used by children with motor or sensory impairments [7]. There is a diverse range of technologies available and suitable for people with different levels of disabilities and for different ages and demographics that can enable such children to have the freedom to experience their three-dimensional environment.

Studies have also shown that ADCS is effective in helping children with autism spectrum disorder (ASD). It provides these children a feeling of control over their space, and encourages them to explore the "real world," outside of their "own world." While the process for children with ASD is very different from children with neuromotor disabilities, ADCS allows children with ASD to close the gap between their world and the real world by allowing them to have freedom and control over the extent of the interaction, which increases with repeated usage.

ADCS can not only assist disabled people to develop their cognitive and motor skills but can also be useful for assisting users with manipulating their environment. This gives them freedom and greater independence, which has been found to be extremely empowering.

7.2 Features of the ADCS

ADCS can be considered to be in two categories: (i) simulation and (ii) robotic. The simulation ADCS allows users to perceive the world with the help of computer simulations of physical conditions. These range from simple computer games to virtual reality with real-life graphics and audio. The robotics can range from simple remote-controlled toys to humanoids that are semiautonomous. Thus, the cost of ADCS ranges from a few dollars to tens of thousands of dollars.

Although there is a range of options for ADCS, one common and essential factor is that these should appear to be nonthreatening, friendly, and fun to the child. It is important that these should have a toylike appearance so that the child is naturally inclined to use them. It is also important to consider the demographics and gender of the child when selecting the ADCS, and factors such as the color and feel of these are also important.

Another important factor for the effectiveness of the ADCS is the speed and complexity of the operations. If the speed and complexity of the device are not matched to the child user, the device will not be very effective. If the response is too fast, the child tends to get threatened, while if it is too slow, the child gets bored and frustrated. There are large and significant differences between different children and thus it is important for the ADCS to allow the user to easily adjust and calibrate the speed of operation in accordance with the needs of the child. Ideally, the ADCS should be dynamic and adaptive such that it identifies the capabilities and needs for the child automatically.

When selecting the suitable ADCS, the child should be carefully assessed prior to the procurement because when the child with disabilities loses interest with the device, it can become significantly more difficult to rekindle his/her interest. Matching the needs of the child with the range of available technologies can often require broad medical and engineering knowledge and thus, engaging the ADCS with experts is useful.

7.3 ADCS Interface

Children who have impaired motor or sensory abilities are unable to use standard interface techniques such as a joystick, computer mouse, or keyboard. This may be due to their inability to have the motor drive perform the action, an inability to feel the pressure and get the feedback, or simply a lack of coordination. The effective use of the ADCS requires the user to easily and surely give the command signal. For this purpose, it is important that the interface should be simplified and its complexity should be suitable for the user.

There are a number of options for developing the interface for the ADCS. There are two aspects of the interface: (i) the command sensor and (ii) the actuator. The sensor is activated by the user to command the device, while the actuator is used to give feedback to the user. The sensors range from a modified computer mouse, accelerometer-based interfaces, and video analysis to eye gaze measurement, brain wave motor imagery, and emotion response measurement methods. While some of these are simply the modification of commercially available systems, such as the Kinect computer game interface for measuring body movement or the use of mobile phones to measure movement, the brain wave measurement systems are very specific and special purpose.

Actuators are required to give feedback to users who are unable to sense the commonly used methods that are based on touch and pressure. These can range from the use of vibration or electrical pulses to visual or audio stimulation.

7.4 Measuring the Success of ADCS

It is important to determine the effectiveness of the ADCS for each child because of the large differences between different children. The success of the ADCS for children with disabilities is not only based on the physical measurements but is also based on the emotional aspects. For this purpose, the "Goal Attainment Scale" (GAS) is one such method [9]. This method gives a numerical measure that combines the physical and emotional outcomes and can be used for ongoing monitoring of the progress of the child, or for the purpose of comparing different ADCSs. GAS also allows the inclusion of subjective evaluations by other people such as parents, teachers, and caretakers who are able to evaluate improvements in the cognitive aspects of the child. It allows the flexibility of defining weights for different aspects such as the attainment of the goal, allows for positive and negative scoring, and can be tailored to the specific child's condition. The global grade is calculated according the grades obtained for all goals accomplished, taking into account the goal accomplished by the child, the number of goals accomplished for each task, and using a constant value to estimate the correlation between the grade and the several goals in the tasks. The global grade is given by [9]

$$T = 50 + 10 \left(\frac{\sum\limits_{i=1}^{n} g_i}{\sqrt{n - Rn + Rn^2}} \right), \tag{7.1}$$

where g_i is the grade related to the goal i accomplished by the child; n is the number of goals accomplished for each task (one task can have several goals, and the partial accomplishment is also taken into account); and R is a constant used to estimate the correlation between the grade and the several goals in the tasks. A constant of $R = 0.3$ is used, as proposed by [8].

Thus, it is possible to evaluate the progress and compare the effectiveness of different ADCS, making it possible to evaluate improvement in terms of learning and grades (which measure how many goals are accomplished), thus having a way to measure the cognitive improvement of the child.

A good ADSC should automatically generate the reports at the end of the experiment. This should have the name, age, gender, and other relevant information of the child; the details of the experiments; the history of selection of the tasks; duration taken by the child for performing each task; the number of movements required to complete the experiment; and a comparison with previous attempts by the same child and by other children.

7.5 Examples of ADCS

7.5.1 Two-Dimensional Path Tracing Computer Simulation

Computer-simulation-based ADSCs have the advantage that these can be generated without requiring any hardware other than a computer with suitable graphics. With the availability of computer tablets and laptops, these have become very inexpensive. One example is shown in

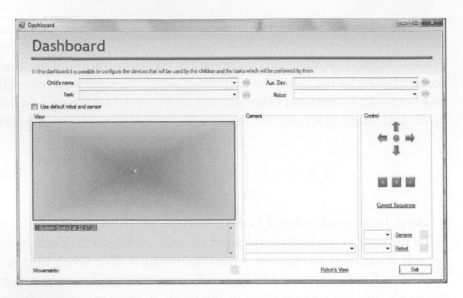

FIGURE 7.1
Main screen of the system. See color insert.

Figure 7.1, where the child has to move to a goal, and this may be done with multiple modalities such as sEMG, accelerometer, or eye gaze. The child's name, robot, and task get registered in the software database. The clinician evaluates each of these, and the system generates reports for each experiment, which helps identify the most suitable modality. It also provides regular progress for the child. The software also has an inbuilt "user assist" that helps the user who may find the task too difficult. This is to ensure that the child continues to be engaged with the ADSC.

7.5.2 Friendly Robot for Children with Motor Disabilities

There are a number of options, and these should be considered for the individual child and circumstances. One example that was used in UFES/Brazil was a mobile robot with tweezers (Pob-Eye, from Pob Technology), which allows the child to use it for sensing and also as a manipulator robot.

The first alteration performed on the original robot was to change the appearance to make it more attractive to children. A simple, handmade clown mask was adapted to the robot, as shown in Figure 7.2. This robot was commanded by the children with limited motor skills. The benefit of this ADSC was the flexibility and diversity of the tasks that the

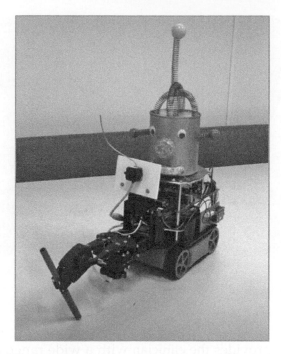

FIGURE 7.2
Mobile robot used in the experiments.

children could be asked to perform while focusing on their interaction with their environment. Some of the tasks were to follow a path, avoid obstacles, and reach a destination where no path was marked, and for manipulation, drawing on a paper using the pen held by the robot.

The mobile robot was commanded by these children using a wireless three-dimensional accelerometer that was worn on their cap (Figure 3.4, Chapter 3), making it suitable for being used by children with cerebral palsy who have no motor control of their hands. Such an interface was found to be reliable, easy to obtain, and did not require any wiring. Another option was the use of myoelectric signal (sEMG) recorded from the forehead and used to identify the eye blinks. Yet another easy-to-implement option is the use of electrooculogram (EOG) recorded from the side of the eyes, which would identify the gaze of the child and make the robot follow the direction of the gaze. These techniques not only allowed the children to control the ADSC but also gave them active feedback, and this empowered them to explore their environment.

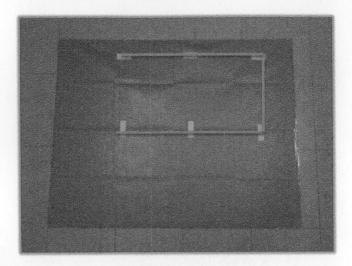

FIGURE 7.3
Drawing a path with the robot.

The ADSC provides the clinician with a wide range of options for helping the child. Some of the tasks that the child can perform using the mobile robot are:

- Task #1: Drawing with the robot. In this case, the robot has a pen held by the tweezers and the child could command the robot to move on a paper in order to draw lines (Figure 7.3).
- Task#2: Free drawing using the mobile robot (Figure 7.4).

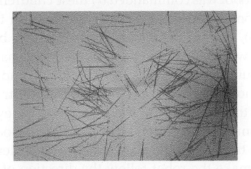

FIGURE 7.4
Free drawing made by a child with disabilities.

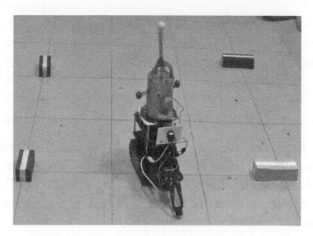

FIGURE 7.5
Obstacle avoidance task.

- Task #3: Command the robot with a briefly defined path to avoid obstacles and reach a destination. In this case, the path contains some color blocks used as obstacles. The free space to move the robot can be reduced, which requires the child to have more accurate movement control (Figure 7.5).

Several trials were carried out with 14 disabled children and it was possible to evaluate the results based on aspects like time to finish the task, total number of movements executed by the child, number and percentage of movements that produce robot movements (valid movements), and movements per second. This evaluation was carried out after several weeks in order to find the improvements obtained with the use of the robot to aid these disabled children.

From these aspects, movements per second and percentage of valid movements seem to represent the more important ones, because the number of movements per second tends to diminish according to the repetition of movements with the robot made by the child. In fact, the number of movements per second decreased 10.6 percent from the first to the third week. In relation to the percentage of valid movements, there was an increase of 4 percent in this parameter after three weeks, which it is expected due to the confidence of using the robot by the children.

Based on these results, it was possible to change and create new tasks in order to try to make those children interact even more with the environment, bringing them more independence and self-esteem. This system also helps the execution of movements by these children in the field of physiotherapy because children feel stimulated to move parts of their body when they realize that their movements can command a robot.

7.5.3 Friendly Robot for Children with Autism Spectrum Disorder (ASD)

A mobile robot can also be used as an ADSC by children with ASD. In that case, the mobile robot is used to allow interaction with these children due to among the characteristics associated with ASD stand out social deficit, deficits in communication and in the production and perception of affective expressions [10] [11].

ASD includes Autism, Asperger Syndrome and Pervasive Developmental Disorder Not Otherwise Specified, with variations in severity and nature of symptoms [12] [13]. The pervasive developmental disorder not otherwise specified and the autism include conditions that may or not be associated with mental retardation [16]. Autism signs are the difficulty in talking about personal feelings and understand the feelings of others, lack of engagement in interactive games, lack of eye contact and joint attention, communication difficulties and sensitivity to physical contact [13]. Asperger syndrome is characterized by deficits in social interaction and the limitation of interests and behaviors, but is differentiated in its early development by the absence of delay in spoken or in perception, cognitive development, self-help skills and in curiosity about the environment [14]. The prevalence of ASD is estimated between 1 and 6 children in 1000, while the prevalence of autism comprises an average of 5.2 per 10,000 children, varying according to the determination of the case [15]. The etiology of ASD is not yet specified, but is probably related to multifactorial conditions of genetic and nongenetic causes (environmental and biological) [16] [17]. Individuals belonging to this spectrum have difficulties in performing independent functions in many important areas of social and occupational life [10]. Currently, there is no cure for this condition, but there are behavioral treatments that can improve the quality of life and independence of individuals with ASD [13] [18].

Beyond human intervention, not human intervention, as social robotics, has been used as a tool for therapy of social and communication skills of children with ASD [10] [19]. Furthermore, the social robotic allows to establish situations of meaningful and sophisticated interaction, using speech, sound, motion and visual indications [18]. Many studies show that the interaction between children with ASD and robots aids the interaction with parents, caretakers and other humans, for example, when the child shows excitement in contact with the robot and turns to one of the parents, expressing his/her excitement [10] [20]. There are also studies that say that interaction with mobile robots has been satisfactory for children with ASD, because robots are predictable, simple and easy to understand [19].

In order to evaluate the impact of using the mobile robot to interact with children with ASD, the following evaluation scales are used: GAS, Fitts' Law and SUS (system usability scale). GAS was previously used in this Chapter to evaluate the performance of children with motor disability when interacting with a mobile robot. On the other hand, the Fitts' Law [21] is used to forecast the necessary time for that a robot movement occurs towards a target area in function of distance and target size, and the system usability scale (SUS) [22] consists of a questionnaire that is used as an tool for evaluate how the child caretaker perceives the usability of the robot to interact with the child. This scale measures aspects such as efficacy (whether the child can successfully achieve their goals), efficiency (how much effort and resources were spent to achieve these goals), and satisfaction (whether the experience in achieving those goals was satisfactory). Thus, the purpose of using these scales is to evaluate the interaction between children with ASD and the mobile robot, in addition to evaluate the robot movement and its usability and efficiency in stimulating social interaction skills of these children, such as eye contact and attention.

The mobile robot used was the PIONNER 3-AT, in which a camera (to capture the child face) and a display and a sound system for the issuance of images and sounds were attached to it in order to attract the child's attention (Figure 7.6. Moreover, the robot also has a laser sensor for the automatic detection and location of the child's position, so that it can establish a minimum safe distance. Thus, the robot approaches and goes away itself from the child, sending images and sounds and allowing the beginning of an interaction.

Table 7.1 describes the levels of attainment for two goals evaluated in the process of interaction between the child with ASD and the robot. A numerical value is assigned for each activity performed, with 0 indicating the expected level of performance and −2 and +2 indicating the least and most favorable results, respectively.

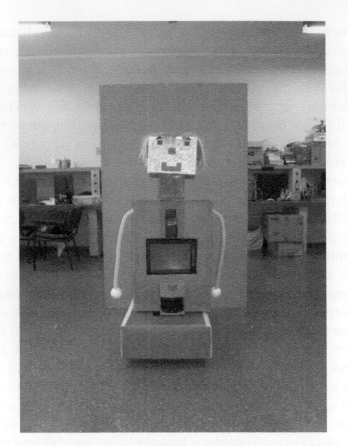

FIGURE 7.6
Mobile robot PIONNER 3-AT and its ludic image.

Another method of interaction analysis consists of a behavioral assessment of the child with ASD, which takes into account the emotional state of the child at the moment of the interaction with the robot. For this, the opinion of the team of psychologist, pedagogue, teachers and caretaker involved with the child with ASD is considered.

To assess the precision of the robot motion towards the child, referring to the moment it takes to attract his/her attention, the Fitts' Law is used, whose accuracy depends on both the distance between child and robot and the size of a target. The time for a motion (MT) is given by [23] [24]:

$$MT = a + b.log_2(D/W), \tag{7.2}$$

where a and b are constants, D is the distance from the starting position to the target center, W is the target width.

TABLE 7.1

Goal Attainment Scaling for Two Goals.

Predict Attainment	Score	Goal 1: Look at the robot	Goal 2: Touch the robot
Most unfavorable outcome	−2	Look at the robot for less than 30 s and present repulsion	Do not touch the robot
Less than expected outcome	−1	Look at the robot for less than 30 s and no interest	Touch the robot for less than 5 s
Expected level of outcome	0	Look at robot for more than 30 s and maintain eye contact	Touch the robot for more than 5 s
Greater than expected outcome	1	Look at the robot for more than 30 s and present joint attention	Touch the robot for more than 5 s and play with it
Most favorable outcome likely	2	Look at the robot for more than 30 s and go towards it	Touch the robot for more than 5 s and present joint attention

On the other hand, to measure and classify the ease of use (usability) of the mobile robot as possible interactive tool for children with ASD, the System Usability Scale (SUS) is used. SUS consists of ten items, where even-numbered items worded negatively, and odd-numbered items worded positively. The caretaker evaluates the robot using 5-point scales numbered from 1 ("Strongly disagree") to 5 ("Strongly agree"), where the number 3 means the center of the rating scale (if the caretaker fails to respond to an item). The items are [25]:

1. I think that I would like to use this system frequently.
2. I found the system unnecessarily complex.
3. I thought the system was easy to use.
4. I think that I would need the support of a technical person to be able to use this system.
5. I found the various functions in this system were well integrated.
6. I thought there was too much inconsistency in this system.

7. I would imagine that most people would learn to use this system very quickly.
8. I found the system very cumbersome to use.
9. I felt the system very confident using the system.
10. I needed to learn a lot of things before I could get going with this system.

The contribution for the items' values ranges from 0 to 4 (being 4 the most positive answer). For odd items (worded positively), subtract 1 from the value given by the user, and for the even items (worded negatively) subtract 5 from the value given by the user. Then, the scores are added and multiplied by 2.5 to get the overall value, ranging from 0 to 100. Normally, in SUS, values above 68 are considered above average, while values below 68 are below average [22].

Thus, the use of the mobile robot can trigger a positive interaction with the child, i.e., stimulate attention and movement of the child with ASD as well as the ability to interact with the environment and people around them. Therefore, these scales are efficient methods of assessment to ensure the robot's utility and safety in interactions with the child with ASD.

GAS allows quantifying the subjective evaluation of the interaction between the child with ASD and the robot. On the other hand, the association of behavioral and emotional analysis of the child, together to GAS, performed by professionals, unleashes a more effective analysis of the process of interaction between the child with ASD and the robot. Also, Fitts' law provides efficiently an assessment of the accuracy of the robot motion to that the child's safety and integrity are preserved at the moment of interaction between child and robot. Finally, in order to evaluate the use of the mobile robot as a pedagogical tool in the treatment of children with ASD, SUS attends efficiently due to it is a highly robust and versatile evaluation scale for the usefulness of the robot.

References

[1] R M Thomas, *Comparing Theories of Child Development*. Wadsworth Publishing, 3a ed., Belmont, CA, 1992.

[2] T W Linder, *Transdisciplinary Play-Based Assessment; Functional Approach to Working with Young Children*. Baltimore, PH Brooks, 1990.

[3] A M Cook, K Howery, *Robot-Enhanced Discovery and Exploration for Very Young Children with Disabilities*. International Technology and Persons with Disabilities Conference, 1998.

[4] R P Brinker, M Lewis, *Discovering the Competent Disabled Infant: a Process Approach to Assessment and Intervention*. Topics in Early Childhood Spec. Educ., Vol. 2(2), pp. 1–15, 1982.

[5] A L Scherzer, I Tscharnuter, *Early Diagnosis and Therapy in Cerebral Palsy*. Marcel Dekker, 2nd ed., New York, 1990.

[6] B Todia, L K Irvin, G H S Singer, P Yovanoff, *The Self-Esteem Parent Program. Disability, and Empowerment Families*. Singer GHS & Powers LE (eds), Toronto, Paul H Brookes, 1993.

[7] Y Swinth, D Anson, J Deitz, *Single-Switch Computer Access for Infants and Toddlers*. American Journal of Occupation Therapy, Vol. 47 (11), pp. 1031–1038, 1993.

[8] A M Cook, B Bentz, N Harbottle, C Lynch, B Miller, *School-Based Use of a Robotic Arm System by Children with Disabilities*. IEEE Trans Neural Systems and Rehabilitation Engineering, Vol. 13(4), pp. 452–460.

[9] T J Kiresuk, A Smith, J E Cardillo, *Goal Attainment Scaling: Applications, Theory and Measurement*. Hillsdale, NJ: Erlbaum, 1994.

[10] E S Kim, L D Berkovits, E P Bernier, D Leyzberg, F Shic, R Paul, B Scassellati, *Social Robots as Embedded Reinforcers of Social Behavior in Children with Autism*. J Autism Dev Disord., vol.43, pp. 1038–1049, 2013.

[11] B Robins, F Amirabollahian, Z Ji, K Dautenhahn, *Tactile Interaction with a Humanoid Robot for Children with autism: A Case Study Analysis Involving User Requirements and Results of an Initial Implementation*. RO-MAN, IEEE, pp. 704–711, 2010.

[12] D A Rossignol, R E Frye, *Mitochondrial Dysfunction in Autism Spectrum Disorders: a Systematic Review and Meta-Analysis*. Molecular Psychiatry, vol. 17, pp. 290–314; 2012.

[13] B Scassellati, H Admon, M Mataric, *Robots for Use in Autism Research*. Annu. Rev. Biomed. Eng, vol. 14, pp. 275–94, 2012.

[14] A Klin, *Autism and Asperger Syndrome: an Overview*. Rev Bras Psiquiatr, vol. 28, supl. I, pp. S3–11, 2006.

[15] World Health Organization (WHO), *Weekly Epidemiological Record*, vol. 78 (4), pp. 17–24, 2003.

[16] M. Rutter, *Aetiology of Autism: Findings and Questions*. Journal of Intellectual Disability Research, vol. 49 (4), pp. 231–238, 2005.

[17] R C Campos, *Neurological Aspects of Infantile Autism*. Pervasive Developmental Disorders: 3rd Millennium, 2nd ed., vol. 2. Brasilia: CORDE, pp. 21–23, 2005.

[18] F Michaud, A Clavet, *Robotoy Contest-Designing Mobile Robotic Toys for Autistic Children*. Proceedings of the American Society for Engineering Education (ASEE'01), 2001.

[19] A Duquette, F Michaud, H Marcier, *Exploring the Use of a Mobile Robot as an Imitation Agent with Children with Low-Functioning Autism*. Auton Robot, vol. 24, pp. 147–157, 2007.

[20] H Kozima, M P Michalowski, C Nakagawa, *Keepon: a Playful Robot for Research, Therapy and Entertainment*. International Journal of Social Robotics, vol. 1, no.1, pp. 3–18, 2009.

[21] I S MacKenzie, *Fitts' Law as a Research and Design Tool in Human-Computer Interaction*. Journal Human-Computer Interaction, vol. 7 (1), pp. 91–139, 1992.

[22] J Brooke, *SUS: a Retrospective*. Journal of Usability Studies, vol. 8, issue 2, 2013.

[23] P M Fitts, J R Peterson, *Information Capacity of Discrete Motor Responses*. Journal of Experimental Psychology, vol. 67 (2), pp. 103–112, 1964.

[24] N J Ferrier, *Achieving a Fitts Law Relationship for Visual Guided Reaching*. Sixth International Conference on Computer Vision, pp.903–910, 1998.

[25] J R Lewis, J Sauro, *The Factor Structure of the System Usability Scale*. Human Centered Design. Lecture Notes in Computer Science, vol. 5619, pp. 94–103, 2009.

8

Upper-Limb Prosthetic Devices

Sridhar Poosapadi Arjunan and Dinesh Kant Kumar
RMIT University, Australia

Leandro Bueno, John Villarejo-Mayor, and Teodiano Freire Bastos-Filho
Universidade Federal do Espírito Santo, Brazil

CONTENTS

8.1 Introduction

Upper limbs have a very important role for humans that is not limited to physical/functional activities but is also intimately linked with psychosocial roles, including looks, and for communication, gestures, control, and sensation. Forearm amputation is devastating and changes the lives of the sufferers.

Limb loss is a major cause of hardship for people around the globe, and people in countries that have fewer resources seem to suffer more than people in the developed world. In the United States, about

1.7 million people live with limb loss and approximately 185,000 amputation-related hospital discharges occur annually [4]. In recent years, trauma-related amputations have decreased compared to disease-related amputations, but they still constitute the majority of upper-limb amputations [5]. Usually, young, active, and economically productive people are affected by traumatic amputations [6]. Upper-limb traumatic amputations occur twice as frequently as traumatic amputations of lower limbs [5] [7].

To provide support for the patients, hand and arm prostheses were developed during the past thousand years. While the earlier versions were simple mechanical hooks that were operated by the user and that allowed the user to push or pull, later developments led to devices that had greater functionality such as gripping an object, and there were also the cosmetic versions that were nonfunctional but restored the look. Recent advancements have resulted in the current electrically powered prosthesis that provide a high degree of freedom and also incorporate the cosmetic look of the hand, carefully matched with the skin texture and size of the user. A prosthetic hand is an important part of the rehabilitation process for hand amputees and requires a better functional movement suitable for the users.

8.1.1 History

Upper-limb prosthetic devices have a long history of development from their primitive stages to the present highly functional and cosmetic prosthetic hands. Until about 1000 CE there was not much advancement in the upper-limb prosthesis, which consisted of a hook that was operated by a combination of ropes operated by the user [2] [3] [12].

The period between the 14th and 18th centuries proved to be a boom for prosthetic devices due to advancements in medical discoveries, and perhaps fueled by wars with European engagement. During this period, the devices were improved due to the availability of novel materials of the time, and these were generally made of copper, iron, wood (Figure 8.1), and steel. Many of these devices were made to conceal the deformities or injuries sustained in the war or due to disease [2] [3].

The biggest spurt in the development of prosthetic hands took place soon after World War II. Post–World War II, there was a demand for improvement in the devices from the war veterans due to the increase in

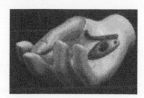

FIGURE 8.1
Prosthetic hand made of wood [3].

soldiers returning from the war with injuries, social pressures, and the availability of excess manufacturing facilities and new materials that had been developed during the war. Thus, these devices could be mass-produced, and the availability of aluminum and plastics made these lighter and more durable. However, there was a lack of technology for such devices and this paved the way for research, development, and improvement in the function of the prosthetic devices. This resulted in devices that are much lighter and stronger, and made with a range of materials such as plastics, metals, and aluminum and composite materials, providing greater functionality [2] [3]. Table 8.1 shows various types of upper-limb prosthesis.

8.2 Prosthetic Hands

Prosthetic hands have been rapidly advancing in recent years with the goal of providing simultaneous, independent, and proportional control of multiple degrees of freedom. When choosing a prosthesis, the following points have to be considered: (i) the level of amputation, (ii) contour of the residual limb, (iii) expected function of the prosthesis, (iv) cognitive function of the user, (v) nature of the job of the user, (vi) hobbies of the user, (vii) cosmetic importance of the prosthesis, and (viii) financial resources of the user [5] [8] [13]. The prosthetic hand devices can be divided into two major types: passive or active, as detailed in the next section.

8.2.1 Passive Prosthetic Devices

Passive prosthetic devices that have no movement in the parts are generally used for cosmetic purposes. These passive prosthetic hands

TABLE 8.1

Various Types of Upper-Limb Prosthesis.

Type	Advantages	Disadvantages
Cosmetic	Most lightweight, best cosmetics, less harnessing	High cost if custom made, least function, low cost glove stains easily
Body powered	Moderate cost, moderately lightweight, most durable, highest sensory feedback, variety of prehensors available for various activities	Requires body movement which may be complex, requires uncomfortable harness, unsatisfactory appearance, increased energy expenditure
Battery powered (myoelectric and/or switch controlled)	Moderate or no harnessing, least body movement needed to operate, moderate cosmetics, more function- proximal areas, stronger grasp in some cases	Heaviest, most expensive, high maintenance, limited sensory feedback, extended therapy time for training
Hybrid (cable to elbow or TD and battery powered)	All-cable excursion to elbow or TD	Battery-powered TD weights forearm (harder to lift but good for elbow disarticulation or long THA)
If excursion to elbow and battery-powered TD	All-cable excursion to elbow	Lower pinch for TD and least cosmetic
If excursion to TD and battery-powered elbow	Increased TD pinch, all-cable excursion to TD, low effort to position TD, low-maintenance TD	

TD = Terminal Device; THA = Transhumeral Amputation
Source: (see [1].)

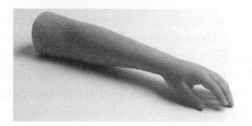

FIGURE 8.2
Passive function prosthetic hand [16].

(Figure 8.2) closely resemble the natural hand and are primarily for aesthetic rather than functional features. With current technology, passive devices can appear remarkably natural and lifelike, matching the skin tone and contours of the person's natural limb [5] [8] [12]. These devices, besides being cosmetic, also provide some important functional abilities to the user, such as pushing, balancing, and supporting. These devices are being termed *passive functional prosthetic devices* [12].

Since passive prostheses do not have any electronic or mechanically powered moving parts, they are lighter in weight compared with active devices. Livingskin prosthesis (Touchbionics, UK) [16] is an example of the currently available state-of-the art passive devices. This passive terminal device has been designed to look more lifelike (Figure 8.2). It is hand crafted from high-definition silicone and hand painted to match the skin tone and appearance of the user. In addition to its realistic appearance, it also provides some important functional capabilities, such as pushing, pulling, stabilizing, supporting, light grasping, and typing [9].

Some of the important features of this device are (i) adjustable finger shape, (ii) skin color located underneath the outer layer, and (iii) silicone material. The advantages of these devices are (i) they can be fitted with adjustable armatures to allow prepositioning of each finger for specific tasks, (ii) the skin color and other features are beneath the outer clear silicone layer to prevent fading, (iii) the silicone material provides a versatile, durable, and virtually stain-proof prosthetic option [9].

8.2.2 Active Prosthetic Devices

Active prosthetic devices are categorized into *body-powered* or *externally powered* devices. A body-powered prosthesis uses harness and cables where various terminal devices like hooks and hands can be attached. These have the advantage of simple operational mechanisms, easy maintenance, moderate cost, and reliability. However, these have highly limited functionalities and are currently used in societies that are economically challenged, lack high-tech maintenance capabilities, and have simpler medical and rehabilitation resources.

The externally powered prosthetic devices use electric, pneumatic, or hybrid power systems. Advances in biomedical engineering have resulted in myoelectric (stump muscle activity) based control being most commonly used for controlling these prosthetic devices. The input signals to control these devices are based on the Myoelectric signal (sEM) generated by the muscle activation of the residual muscles. Such prosthetic hand devices have been improving since the 1960s when these were first introduced [5]. Below is a brief description of the various technologies.

8.2.2.1 Body-Powered Prosthestic Hand

The prosthesis that is powered by the power of the body can use a combination of forces generated by the person, typically from the combination of the shoulder and the other hand. The challenges in the design of these devices have been the reliability, the ability of the user to control the device effectively, and safety, which may be compromised due to slippage and unintended loosening.

In earlier days, Bowden cable control systems were one of the most successful and commonly used control systems for body-powered prosthetic devices. This system uses the motions and force generated by the movement of the body to actuate and control a mechanical terminal device such as the prosthetic hand, shown in Figure 8.3. One important advantage of this type of control is that it naturally provides a degree of sensory feedback related to force and position. However, this requires an adequate degree of force and body extension to actuate and control the upper-limb mechanical terminal device [5] [8] [14] [15].

The main advantages of body-powered devices are (i) lower initial cost, (ii) light weight, (iii) easier to repair, and (iv) direct feedback to the user. The disadvantages of these devices are (i) their appearance with a number of wires, and (ii) their difficulty of use by people who lack strength since it depends on the user's physical ability [5].

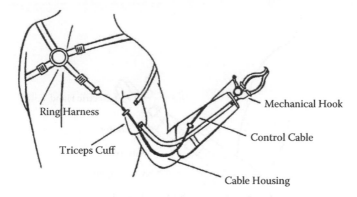

FIGURE 8.3
Bowden cable harness prosthetic control [12].

8.2.2.2 Externally Powered Prosthetic Hand

A prosthetic hand that is operated by external power has a number of advantages for the user because it allows a more natural use of the hand. Several options are possible, such as the use of electrical solenoids, electrical motors, or pneumatics. However, the challenge has been due to the size and weight of these devices and the force that can be provided. The size and weight of these devices has been improving rapidly with the availability of microdevices and new lightweight materials, making powered prosthetic hands a reality.

Another type of externally powered prosthesis is the switch controlled prosthesis, which utilizes small switches rather than muscle signals to operate the electric motors. These switches are enclosed inside the socket or incorporated into the suspension harness of the prosthesis and can be activated by the movement of a remnant digit or part of a bony prominence against the switch or by a pull on a suspension harness. This provides an alternate and viable option to provide control for external power when myoelectric control sites are not available or when the patient cannot master myoelectric control.

Having developed the ability to power hands, the difficulty was in interfacing the device with the patient so that the patient can effectively control these devices. There are number of different options, such as brain neural interface, implantable neuromuscular interface, and electroencephalogram (EEG) based interfaces. Examples such as the brain wave controlled devices are specialdevices for people who do not have

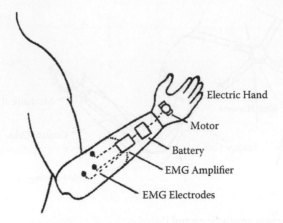

FIGURE 8.4
Myoelectric-based electric-powered devices [12].

any muscle of the hand. These devices are still in the research stage and are perhaps two decades away from commercial reality. However, the most effective and natural prosthesis for people who have the stump muscles of the hand is the use of myoelectric-controlled hands.

8.2.2.3 Myoelectric Prosthetic Control System

Myoelectric control systems measure the electrical activity of the muscle and are an indicator of the strength of muscle contraction. Myoelectric prosthetic hand control is based on the muscle activity of the section of the muscle that is remaining after the amputation. This activity is recorded from the surface of the stump and analyzed after initial amplification and signal processing. This is used to identify the command and control of the battery-powered electromechanical prosthetic device. An example of this kind of prosthesis is shown in Figure 8.4. Another example is UFES's prosthesis, which is shown in Figure 8.5. This upper-limb prosthesis consists of a microcontroller, electronic circuitry to actuate the artificial hand, and the following sensors: myoelectric, temperature, and force and slip. The microcontroller acquires information from sensors and controls the artificial hand and a vibrator inside the prosthesis. Thus, if the temperature is higher than 45°C, the user is alerted by the vibrators, whose amplitude of vibration increases with the temperature; if the temperature is higher than 60°C, the controller prevents the artificial hand from closing. The temperature T is inferred as a function of the voltage provided by KTY

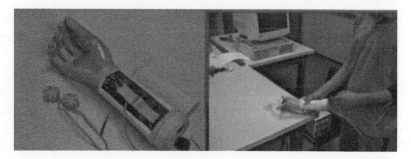

FIGURE 8.5
Myoelectric prosthesis developed in UFES/Brazil, which has force and temperature sensors. See color insert.

temperature sensors attached to hand fingers, given by Equation 8.1. In a grasp operation, if the object starts to slip when it is lifted by the artificial hand, the controller is commanded to increase the force on the object until it stops slipping. The force is inferred as a function of resistance R provided by FSR force sensors also attached to fingers, given by Equation 8.2.

$$T = 84V - 144 \ (^{\circ}\text{C}) \tag{8.1}$$

$$R = 1.3 \times 10^6 F^{-0.9} \ (\Omega) \tag{8.2}$$

The main advantages of these electric-powered prosthetic devices are that they do not require a harness or cable and hence can be built to look more like a real hand. Since they are battery powered, the body strength and movement are not as important for their operation. These devices provide a strong grip force as compared to the body-powered devices [9]–[11].

The disadvantages of using these electric-powered devices are [3] [5] [8]:

- Higher initial cost
- Heavier. However, with lighter and rechargeable batteries, and lighter materials, the weight of these devices has been reduced significantly.
- Higher repair cost. This is largely due to the mechanical failures of the fingers, and the electronic failures due to vibration and moisture. However, improved materials and development of microdevices have significantly improved the reliability and robustness of these devices.

- Dependence on battery life. The improved batteries, improved motor drivers, and availability of rechargeable batteries have overcome this limitation to a large extent.

Some examples of recently available technology in the externally powered hands are the SensorHand by Advanced Arm Dynamics, which has an AutoGrasp feature, an opening/closing speed of up to 300 mm/second, and advanced signal processing techniques, and the i-LimbT hand (Touch Bionics), sometimes referred to as the bionic hand, a commercially available myoelectric hand prosthesis with individually powered digits. There are also individual prosthetic digits for one or more fingers in patients with amputation at a trans-metacarpal level or higher [9].

Pneumatic-powered hands have also been developed for people with shoulder-level amputation and have been used particularly for children. Due to the weight of the body-powered hand, which typically weighs 550 g, a bigger load distribution is introduced on the forearm stump. This becomes hard for children to handle the weight and size of the hand. Pneumatic power can overcome some of these disadvantages since a pneumatic motor is light-weight, fast, and reliable. For example, the electric motor can be replaced by a pneumatic version that weighs less than 2 g and that can be coupled directly to the fingers. The control system is usually by the operation of a valve that is incorporated in a harness. Due to its power recharge problems, the use of harness, and its limited functionality, this system has not been popular among users [14].

The latest technology advancement in the prosthetic hand is to design artificial muscles that can be used to control the individual fingers and provide various complex wrist movements and grip movements. Air Muscles Hand, developed by Shadow Robot Company, is an actuator that is small, light, and simple. It is a linear actuator, producing motion along a straight line and opening a whole new range of design possibilities. These have been called Shadow Air Muscles, and these do not behave identically to the pneumatic cylinder or other linear actuators but provide the functionality of real muscles. As the Air Muscle contracts under constant pressure, pulling force produced between the endpoints decreases. The maximum possible force at a given pressure is obtained when the Air Muscle is stretched out to maximum length.

There are also other technologies that are under development to provide better tactile feedback from the prosthetic hand device to the user. For example, the Smart Hand developed by EU researchers is a complex prosthesis with four motors and 40 sensors designed to provide realistic motion and sense to the user. They have claimed that the Smart Hand is the first prosthetic device to send signals back to the wearers, allowing them to feel what they touch [11] [15].

8.3 Current Prosthetic Devices

Most common commercially available prosthetic hands have been discussed in this section. Most of these devices are battery powered and myoelectric controlled. Some of these devices include ProDigits and i-Limb (Touch Bionics), Bebionic hand, Myobock SensorHand, Otto Bock myoelectric prosthesis (Otto Bock), LTI Boston Digital Arm System (Liberating Technologies, Inc.), ShadowHand, Air Muscles (Shadow Robot Inc.), and the Utah Arm Systems (Motion Control) [14] [15].

8.3.1 User Benefits

The features of these devices are to provide a more natural-looking hand and to move more like a natural hand. Each of these devices has its own unique technology to control the hand where fingers move independently and bend at the natural joints. The i-Limb (Figure 8.6) uses its own unique software to accurately adapt so that it can fit around the shape of the object that needs to be grasped. This myoelectric-based hand is powered by Touch Bionics's unique software with advanced technology, providing the ability to customize the hand for daily needs [9].

A comparison of the current state-of-the-art prosthetic hands shows that most features of these devices are very comparable. However each of these devices also has its unique strengths. For example, i-Limb ultra allows variable digit-by-digit grip strength, the gesture selection allows users to create custom gestures, and its unique *biosim* software allows selection of automatic hand modes, signal assessment, gestures, and training modes [9]. Similarly, the Myobock myoelectric

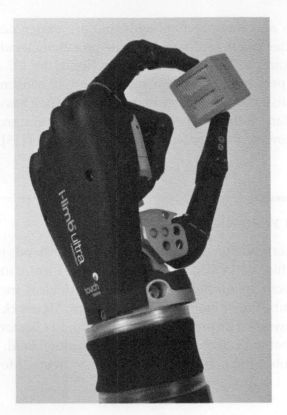

FIGURE 8.6
i-Limb Ultra, Touchbionics,UK [9].

SensorHand has a better grip speed, the ability to control grip speed, and senses the level of control. Most of these devices also have active and natural skin covers to look more lifelike. The i-Limb provides better power management, which extends daily battery usage by 25 percent [9] [11].

i-Limb and Bebionic hands have similar features and have multiple motors that allow for independent control for each finger, and such a hand can grip an object in a natural and coordinated way. The Bebionic hand utilizes leading-edge technology and unique, ergonomic features for better versatility, functionality, and performance. The motors are positioned to optimize weight distribution, making the hand feel lighter and more comfortable [9]–[11].

In terms of the grip strength and the pattern, the Myobock myoelectric SensorHand has a better grip speed and the ability to control grip speed, when compared with other available electric-powered hands. It offers a maximal grip speed of 300 mm/s, which gives better grasp of various objects without much effort. The speed of the SensorHand is easy to control and is precise based on their new intelligent software and modified signal processing. The SensorHand has the ability to sense a change in the center of gravity and readjusts its grip automatically [10] [11].

The most common and important features of these devices are (i) they have five individually powered articulating fingers, (ii) manually rotatable thumb to create different grasping options, (iii) manually rotatable wrist, (iv) proportional control, based on the strength of the input signal, making the fingers move faster, (iv) compatible with a wide range of upper-limb devices and provides better grip force, and (v) they are made of an aluminium chassis that provides more durability and is lighter weight [9]–[11].

When compared with other electrically powered hands, the Bebionic hand has powerful microprocessors that continuously monitor the position of each finger, which gives the user precise and reliable control over hand movements. It has 14 selectable grip patterns and hand positions, more than any other commercially available hand, which enables the user to perform a large number of everyday activities with less difficulty [9]–[11].

One important feature that has been imparted in currently developed hands is proportional control. This proportional speed control provides the user a precision control over delicate tasks, such as picking up an egg or holding a polystyrene cup without crushing them [10] [11].

This prosthetic hand has selectable thumb positions and a built-in sensor that enables the user to complete more tasks and also has an auto-grip feature that provides safety. The durable construction and advanced materials make this Bebionic hand strong. In comparison with other hands, its innovative palm design protects the hand from impact damage and makes the hand quieter when it is used. Its soft finger pads and a wide thumb profile provide maximum surface area and enhance the finger grips [10].

8.3.2 Specifications

Most of the devices have an operating voltage at 7.4 V (nominal) and the maximum current is 5 A. The i-Limb hand has a maximum hand load

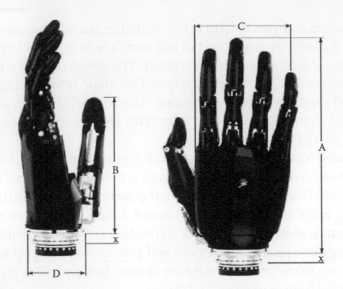

FIGURE 8.7
Myobock system electric hands [10].

limit (static limit) corresponding to 90 kg/198 lb and the finger carry load (static limit) is 32 kg/71 lb. When compared with other similar devices, this hand has greater strength and allows for more natural and normal control for the user. The weight of the i-Limb hand device is 419 g, which is lighter considering other powered devices [9]–[11].

The SensorHand (Figure 8.7) has better proportional speed, which is in the range of 15 to 300 mm/s. This allows the hand to move between different gestures without any delay [11].

References

[1] A Esquenazi, J A Leonard, R H Meier, *Prosthetics, orthotics and assistive devices*. Arch Phys Med Rehabil., Vol. 70 (5-S), pp. S206–209, 1989.

[2] Artificial right hand, *Europe*. http://www.sciencemuseum.org.uk/broughttolife/objects/display.aspx, pp. 1915–1925, accessed Dec 10, 2012.

[3] K N Norton, *A brief history of prosthetics*. in Motion, Vol. 17 (7), pp. 1–4, 2007.

[4] T R Dillingham, L E Pezzin, E J MacKenzie, *Limb amputation and limb deficiency: Epidemiology and recent trends in the United States.* South Med J, Vol. 95 (8), pp. 875–883, 2002.

[5] B M Kelly, *Upper limb prosthetics,* http://emedicine.medscape. com/article/317234-overview, accessed Dec 11, 2012.

[6] A Esquenazi, *Amputation rehabilitation and prosthetic restoration: From surgery to community reintegration.* Disabil Rehabil, Vol. 26 (14–15), pp. 831–836, 2004.

[7] A E Freeland, R Psonak, *Traumatic below-elbow amputations.* Ortho- pedics, Vol. 30 (2), pp. 120–126, 2007.

[8] WorkSafeBC, *Upper limb prostheses: A review of the literature with a focus on myoelectric hands. Evidence-based practice group,* http://www.worksafebc.com/evidence, accessed Nov 20, 2012.

[9] I-limb Ultra, *Touchbionics,* http://www.touchbionics.com/ products/active-prostheses/i-limb-ultra, accessed Dec 10, 2012.

[10] Bebeionic3 hand, http://bebionic.com/the_hand, accessed Dec 10, 2012.

[11] Myobock Electric hands, http://www.ottobock.com/cps/rde/ xchg/ob _com_en/hs.xsl/384.html, accessed Dec 10, 2012.

[12] J N Billock, *Upper limb prosthetic terminal devices: Hands versus hooks,* Clin Prosthet Orthot, Vol. 10 (2), pp. 57–65, 1986.

[13] Prosthetic Devices for Upper-Extremity Amputees, *Military in Step,* http://www.amputee-coalition.org/military-instep/ prosthetic-devices-upper.pdf, accessed July 10, 2013.

[14] L M Kruger, S Fishman, *Myoelectric and body-powered prostheses,* J Pediatr Orthop. Vol. 13 (1), pp. 68–75, 1993.

[15] Medical policy: Myoelectric prosthesis for the upper limb, https://www.premera.com/medicalpolicies/cmi_061275.htm, accessed Dec 10, 2012.

[16] Livingskin, *Touchbionics,* http://www.touchbionics.com/products/ passive-functional-prostheses/livingskin, accessed Dec 10, 2012.

Appendix

Countries with Disability Programs

Dinesh Kant Kumar
RMIT University, Australia

Teodiano Freire Bastos-Filho
Universidade Federal do Espírito Santo, Brazil

CONTENTS

References 194

Table A.1 shows some countries that have one or more disability programs.

TABLE A.1
Example of Countries with Disability Programs

Country	Program	Conditions	Type of disability	Support amount
Australia[1]	Disability Support Pension	Individuals aged between 16 and 64 and are unable to work will be retrained to work for 15 hours or more per week within the next two years.	Permanently blind, or have a physical, intellectual, or psychiatric disability.	Maximum fortnightly payments. Over 21: Single: $733.70. Member of a couple: $553.10 each or $1,106.20 combined. Under 21: Single, under 18, at home: $338.40. Single, under 18, independent: $522.90. Single, 18–20, at home: $383.60. Single, 18–20, independent: $522.90. A member of a couple, up to age 20: $522.90

Brazil[2]	Disability Support Pension	For people with severe disability, benefits will be available after 25 years of contribution for men and 20 years for women. For people with moderate disability, benefits will be available after 29 years of contribution for men and 24 for women. For people with light disability, benefits will be available after 33 years of contribution for men and 28 for women. Since October 2013, the Brazilian government provides a free electric wheelchair for people unable to use a manual wheelchair.	High, moderate, light	Monthly payments variable depending on time of contribution: from R$678,00 to R$4.157,05

continued

TABLE A.1
Example of Countries with Disability Programs *continued*

Country	Program	Conditions	Type of disability	Support amount
Canada[3]	Canada Pension Plan (CPP) Disability Benefit	For people who actively contributed to the plan while working but are now unable to work at any job regularly due to a disability and are below 65 years of age	Disability that is severe and prolonged, preventing the individual from working at any job on a regular basis	Monthly payments variable depending on individual's situation. In 2010 the average CPP disability benefit: $807.81
Canada[4]	Registered Disability Savings Plan	For individuals under 60 years of age. This is to enable people with a disability to save, by contributing 100–300% of the amount saved by the person	Severe and prolonged physically impairment or mentally	Variable dependent on individual's income: Maximum of $3,500 in one year and up to $70,000 over the person's lifetime

| India[5,6] | Assistance to disabled persons for purchase/ fitting of aids and appliances (ADIP Scheme) | Indian citizen certified from a medical practitioner that he/she is physically disabled. Their monthly income cannot exceed Rs. 10,000 and they have not received assistance from other nongovernment agencies in the last three years for the same purpose. Aids/appliances costing less than Rs. 6,000 are covered | Any disability requiring aids/appliances for social, economic, and vocational rehabilition | Funds are allocated district-wise to agencies in charge of implementing the scheme. In 2011–2012, this amount was approximately Rs. 1,150,000. The cost ranges from Rs. 500 for hearing and speech impairment to Rs. 1,000 for the visually disabled and Rs. 3,000 for the orthopedically disabled |

continued

TABLE A.1

Example of Countries with Disability Programs *continued*

Country	Program	Conditions	Type of disability	Support amount
Switzerland[7,8]	Invalidity insurance benefits		Disability that causes an earning incapability that is likely to be permanent or prolonged	Rehabilitation measures to aid in daily activities and improve quality of life, which includes medical measures, supply of aids/appliances, occupational measures, and cash benefits. In 2011, social insurance benefits were $8,529, and the Invalidity insurance pensions were $238,333

| United Kingdom[9] | Disability Living Allowance | Individuals aged under 16 or 65 or over | Individuals with walking difficulties or if they require help to look after themselves for three months and expect to be disabled for at least six months. Or if they have a debilitating disease and life expectancy is less than six months | Weekly Care component: £21–£79.15. Weekly Mobility component: £21–£55.25 |

continued

TABLE A.1

Example of Countries with Disability Programs *continued*

Country	Program	Conditions	Type of disability	Support amount
United Kingdom[10]	Personal Independence Payment from 2013	People aged 16–64 with a disability	Condition or disability that affects daily activities and/or mobility that they have had for at least three months and expect to have for another 9 months. Terminally ill patients with life expectancy less than six months are also eligible	Daily living component paid weekly: £53–£79.15. Weekly Mobility component: £21–£55.25

Spain[11,12]	Permanent Disability Pension	Individuals under 65 years of age	Disability that makes an individual incapable of performing their work, even after medical treatment	Monthly amounts vary depending on degree of disability: €1,145.00–€384.90
Japan[13]	Disability basic pension	Individual must be insured under the National Pension or is aged 60 to 64 and is residing in Japan, or the individual has a permanent disability before the age of 20 years	Any disability involving the hands, blindness, etc.	Disability grade 1: From 2004 onwards this benefit is 993,100 Yen and an additional amount for children. Disability grade 2: From 2004 onwards, this benefit is 794,500 Yen and additional amounts for children

continued

TABLE A.1

Example of Countries with Disability Programs *continued*

Country	Program	Conditions	Type of disability	Support amount
Germany[14]	Long-term care insurance	Individual who demonstrates the need for care and has been insured for a qualifying time period	Insured individuals who require day-to-day care due to a physical, mental, or psychological illness or disability	Services provided: Free nursing care courses for relatives, care allowance for carers, day- and night-time care, nursing aids and appliances, subsidies for equipping the individual's home to facilitate care. Cash benefits: Home care: €235.00–€700.00 depending on category of care. If assistance is provided by professional caregivers, the benefits received by the individual will be €450.00–€1,918.00 depending on the care category. For full in-patient care, basic personal care and household assistance benefits vary between €1023.00 and €1918.00

France[15]	Disability Insurance	Individuals under the legal retirement age of 60–62.	Any type of disability that prevents an individual from earning equal to at least a third of the wage normally paid for the job they were employed in before the onset of their disability	First category: able to perform some activity, calculated as 30% of their annual earnings with maximum benefits paid at €11,109.60. Second category: unable to perform any activity, calculated as 50% of their annual earning with maximum benefits paid at €18,516.00. Third category: persons requiring a daily carer. In 2012, this benefit was €12,989.19

continued

TABLE A.1

Example of Countries with Disability Programs *continued*

Country	Program	Conditions	Type of disability	Support amount
Singapore[16]	Traffic Accident Fund	Singapore citizens or permanent residents with less than $1,300 gross monthly income	Permanent or temporary disability caused by a transport accident	Provides individuals with financial assistance of up to $10,000 within seven years for purchase of aids and equipment
Singapore[17]	Special Assistance Fund	Singapore citizens or permanent residents with less than $1,300 gross monthly income, who cannot afford the equipment necessary for the disabled	Low-income families who cannot afford to purchase aids for the disabled member	One-off subsidy of up to $10,000 for financial assistance in purchasing of aids for the disabled

| Singapore[18] | Assistive Technology Fund | Singapore citizens with disabilities | Family gross monthly income per capita is below $1,500, and children with disabilities are enrolled in a school program, while the adults are currently working or are applying for jobs that may require an assistive technology device | Covers 90% of the cost of the assistive device, and subject to a maximum of $20,000. Subsidized assistive technology devices include: Braille laptops, speech synthesizers, vision aids, hearing aids, magic wand keyboards |

continued

TABLE A.1
Example of Countries with Disability Programs *continued*

Country	Program	Conditions	Type of disability	Support amount
South Korea[19]	Disability Pension	Aged 18 years and older with monthly income less than KRW 551,000 for persons with disabilities with no spouse, and KRW 881,600 for persons with disabilities and with a spouse	Severe disabilities	Basic benefits: 5% of the monthly average income of national pension insured persons for the past three years is paid. In 2012, this value was KRW 91,200. This benefit is not paid to old pension beneficiaries at the age of 65 or older. Extra benefits: Covers all or a part of additional expenses due to a disability. Monthly amount can be KRW 60,000 and KRW 50,000. For persons aged 65 or older, this value is KRW 20,000

	Disability benefits		
Italy[20]	Italian citizens who are disabled and have made contributions to the disability pensions for five years	A person is considered disabled when his earning capacity is reduced to one third	Calculated on the same basis as the old-age pension, which was at least 1.2 times € 480.53 in 2012.

References

[1] Australian Government, Department of Human Services, *Disability support pension*, http://www.humanservices.gov.au/customer/services/centrelink/disability-support-pension, accessed Apr 16, 2013.

[2] Diário Oficial da União, *República Federativa do Brasil, Imprensa Nacional, Brazil*, http://www.in.gov.br/imprensa, accessed May 26, 2013.

[3] Government of Canada, *CPP disability—I Want to Apply*, http://www.servicecanada.gc.ca/eng/isp/cpp/applicant.shtml, accessed May 25, 2013.

[4] Canada Revenue Agency, *RC 4460 registered disability savings plan*, http://www.cra-arc.gc.ca/E/pub/tg/rc4460/, File: rc4460-12e.pdf, accessed May 25, 2013.

[5] Ministry of Social Justice and Empowerment, Govt. of India, *Empowerment of persons with disabilities—Schemes/programmes*, http://socialjustice.nic.in/pdf/adiprel1112.pdf, File: Details of grant released during the year 2011-12 under ADIP, accessed May 25, 2013.

[6] Ministry of Social Justice and Empowerment, Govt. of India, *Empowerment of persons with disabilities—Schemes/programmes*, http://socialjustice.nic.in/pdf/adipsch.pdf, File: Scheme of assistance to disabled persons for purchase/fitting of aids/appliances (ADIP scheme), accessed Apr 29, 2013.

[7] Federal Department of Home Affairs DHA, Federal Social Insurance Office, Switzerland, *Invalidity insurance benefits*, http://www.bsv.admin.ch/themen/iv/00021/03187/index.html?lang=en, accessed Apr 29, 2013.

[8] Federal Department of Home Affairs DHA, Federal Social Insurance Office, Switzerland, *Key data: Invalidity Insurance*, http://www.bsv.admin.ch/dokumentation/zahlen/00093/00426/ index.html?lang=en, accessed Apr 29, 2013.

[9] Gov. UK, *Disability living allowance (DLA)*, https://www.gov.uk/dla-disability-living-allowance-benefit/overview, accessed Apr 8, 2013.

[10] Gov. UK, *Personal independence payment (PIP)*, https://www.gov.uk/pip/overview, accessed Apr 29, 2013.

[11] Gobierno de Espana, Ministerio de Empleo y Seguridad Social, Spain, *Permanent disability pension*, http://www.seg-social.es/Internet_6/Masinformacion/TramitesyGestiones/Pensionde Incapacida45982, accessed Apr 29, 2013.

[12] Gobierno de Espana, Ministerio de Empleo y Seguridad Social, Spain, *Pensioners*, http://www.seg-social.es/Internet_6/Pensionistas/Revalorizacion/Cuantiasminimas2007/30437_6#30437_6, accessed Apr 29, 2013.

[13] Ministry of Health, Labour and Welfare, Japan, *Outline of National Pension Law, August 2004*, http://www.mhlw.go.jp/english/org/policy/dl/p36-37e.pdf, accessed Apr 30, 2013.

[14] Duetsche Sozialversicherung, Germany, *Long-term care insurance*, http://www.deutsche-sozialversicherung.de/en/longterm_care/index.html, accessed Apr 30, 2013.

[15] The French social security system, I- Sickness, maternity, paternity, disability and death branch, B- *Disability Insurance*, http://www.cleiss.fr/docs/regimes/regime_france/an_1.html, accessed Apr 30, 2013.

[16] Centre for Enabled Living, Singapore, *Traffic Accident Fund*, http://www.cel.sg/Schemes__Traffic-Accident-Fund.aspx, accessed May 20, 2013.

[17] Centre for Enabled Living, Singapore, *Special Assistance Fund*, http://www.cel.sg/Schemes_Special-Assistance-Fund.aspx, accessed May 20, 2013.

[18] Ministry of Social and Family Development, Singapore, *Assistive Technology Fund*, http://app.msf.gov.sg/Assistance/AssistiveTechnologyFundATF.aspx, accessed May 20, 2013.

[19] Ministry of Health & Welfare, Seoul Korea, *Disability pension*, http://english.mw.go.kr/front_eng/jc/sjc0108mn.jsp?PAR_MENU_ID=100309&MENU_ID=10030902, accessed May 20, 2013.

[20] International Group Program, Summary of social security and private employee benefits, Italy, *Disability benefits: National Social Insurance Institute (INPS)*, http://www.igpinfo.com/igpinfo/public_documents/ss_summaries/Italy.pdf, pg. 3, accessed May 20, 2013.

Index

Note: Page numbers ending in "e" refer to equations. Page numbers ending in "f" refer to figures. Page numbers ending in "t" refer to tables.

Printed and bound by CPI Group (UK) Ltd, Croydon, CR0 4YY
18/10/2024
01776262-0002